PRAISE FOR *FITNESS FOR*

"Meg Boggs is an icon and the fitness role model we desperat[...] changer for anyone who wants to feel better, get stronger, and [...] fitness without the harmful distraction of diet culture. Let's all say it louder: Fitness has no size."

—Caroline Dooner, bestselling author of *The F*ck It Diet*

"If you're a woman who's sick of being told that your body is too big to be athletic, or that you'll only be able to accomplish tough physical feats if you look like a fitness model, this book is for you. Part memoir, part anti-diet manifesto, and part strength-training guide, *Fitness for Every Body* offers the liberating perspective that your body is capable of so much more than diet culture gives it credit for—from lifting heavy weights to handling challenges like pregnancy and delivery, mental illness, and whatever else life throws at you."

—Christy Harrison, MPH, RD, author of *Anti-Diet*

"Meg is the definition of REAL. This world needs more women like her, who prove that no matter who you are, your body should be celebrated for all that it can do."

—Lauren Fisher, seven-time CrossFit Games
athlete and founder of Grown Strong

"As a long-time follower of Meg, I feel as though I've gotten a front-row seat at her evolution in the last couple of years. I've learned from her, been in awe of her, and just truly fell in love with her ability to break through barriers and hate when it comes to her fitness and her body.

With *Fitness for Every Body* Meg helps peel that journey back a bit, taking you through facts, combined with experience, that relate to anyone of any size. She uses her story to vehicle a message that everyone needs to hear, learn from, and be empowered by. I think this book is especially important for anyone who lives with thin privilege to identify and dismantle the systems that cause so much fatphobia and weight stigma in our society and learn how we can collectively be a better support to ALL bodies.

This is the book I would pass down to my children to read. I would be honored if my kids would have a woman like Meg Boggs to aspire to."

—Sarah Nicole, blogger at The Birds Papaya

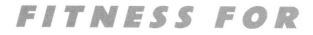

FITNESS FOR

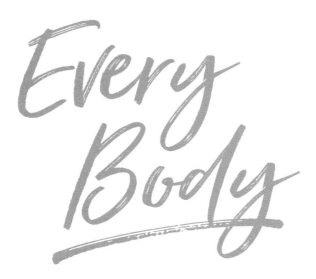

Every Body

STRONG, CONFIDENT,
AND EMPOWERED AT ANY SIZE

MEG BOGGS

ILLUSTRATIONS BY
STEPHANIE CHINN ART

TILLER PRESS

NEW YORK   LONDON   TORONTO   SYDNEY   NEW DELHI

TILLER PRESS

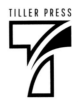

An Imprint of Simon & Schuster, Inc.
1230 Avenue of the Americas
New York, NY 10020

First Tiller Press trade paperback edition April 2021

TILLER PRESS and colophon are trademarks of Simon & Schuster, Inc.

For information about special discounts for bulk purchases, please contact Simon & Schuster Special Sales at 1-866-506-1949 or business@simonandschuster.com.

The Simon & Schuster Speakers Bureau can bring authors to your live event. For more information or to book an event, contact the Simon & Schuster Speakers Bureau at 1-866-248-3049 or visit our website at www.simonspeakers.com.

Interior design by Laura Levatino
Illustrations by Stephanie Chin Art

Manufactured in the United States of America

1   3   5   7   9   10   8   6   4   2

Library of Congress Cataloging-in-Publication Data has been applied for.

ISBN 978-1-9821-5707-4
ISBN 978-1-9821-5708-1 (ebook)

For my daughter, Maci.

And for all the fitness warriors who deserve more representation.

CONTENTS

PART 1: The Part Where We Introduce Ourselves 1

PART 2: The Part Where We Talk about How
Thinness and Fitness Are Not the Same Thing 11

PART 3: The Part Where We Give Moms a Freakin' Break 35

PART 4: The Part Where We Embrace Fitness as We Are 65

PART 5: The Part Where We Pick Up Some Weights 93

PART 6: The Part Where We Remember Our Worth 181

Additional Resources 191

Acknowledgments 203

Notes 205

FITNESS FOR EVERY BODY

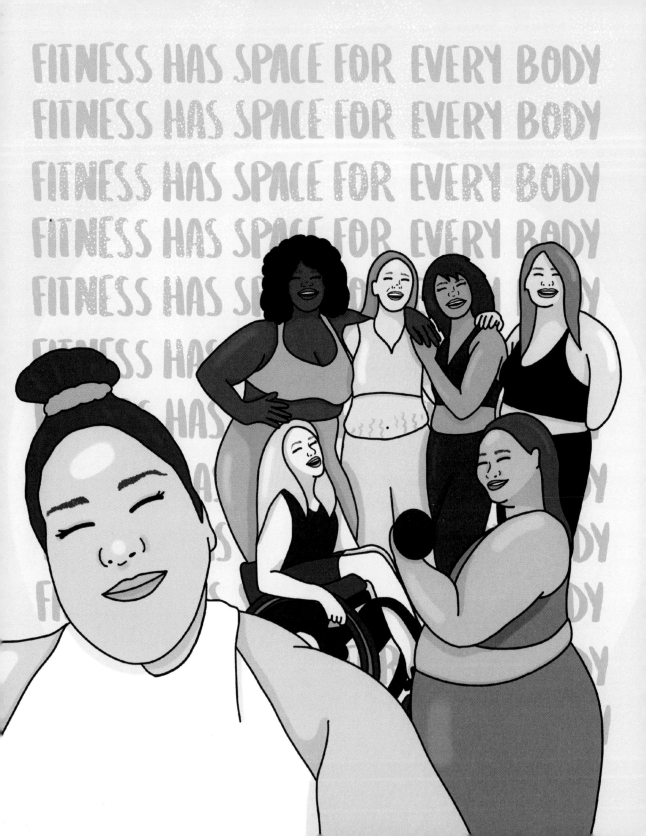

PART 1

The Part Where We Introduce Ourselves

WHY I'M WRITING THIS

First, *breathe*. Sometimes everything gets so overwhelming that we forget this simple practice. So, let's breathe; let's breathe deeply, meaningfully, and with a big "hell yes" as you exhale all of those old, toxic thoughts that convinced you to do uncomfortable things to your body so others could be more comfortable around you. Because it's about time we stop feeling so fucking uncomfortable. So, breathe. *Whew*. Doesn't that feel better?

Now we can start: Hi, I'm Meg. I'm just your average full-of-emotion thirtysomething, living in Texas, trying to stay positive among all the chaos that comes with life's twists and turns. I'm a woman, wife, and mother who happens to be plus-size and is kinda-sorta-basically obsessed with fitness.

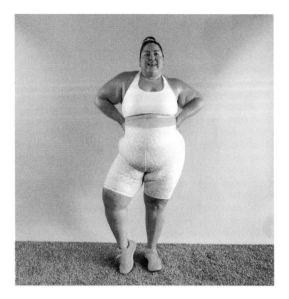

I'm not the transformational weight-loss story you might be used to seeing when bodies like mine are acknowledged in fitness. And that's exactly why I wrote this book.

Even though I've called myself a lot of different things during my life, only about a year ago did I start referring to myself as an athlete. I changed it in my Instagram bio and everything, so it's pretty serious, and I finally feel proud to call myself that. (Because it's exactly what I am.) It's taken a while to start calling myself that. I've spent my life in a body that hasn't been accepted by society, and that hasn't been easy. I've fallen into the deep pits of diet-culture hell. I've clawed my way out of depression multiple times (and counting). I've faced my fears and failed. I've faced my fears and soared gloriously. I've believed all the myths and false truths about fitness and fatness and everything in between. But living through all these experiences has taught me so much. I've self-discovered in ways that I never thought possible, and it has changed my life. I wish I could say that it was because of a formula that I learned, a method that I could then share with you. I don't know the formula. I don't even know if there is a formula. But I'll be damned if I don't try to pick apart the pieces of what I've found and share it with you, because I wish that someone had shared their "formula" with me.

Like every little girl, I had dreams for myself when I was younger. Sometimes I imagined myself on a stage. Other times I imagined myself winning a championship. The dreams felt endless. But at some point, I grew up and I suddenly understood that my dreams were not endless, that they were not achievable, that they would only ever be dreams. And not because of lack of talent or ability, but instead, because of lack of approval. I realized that the body I was born in might not be the body given permission to live fearlessly toward dreams. I can still feel the sun's heat on my face and the wall of my middle school pressed roughly against my back, as I sat on the dirt, devastated after being called "fat." My bullies' roaring laughter has burned itself into my memory. I can still feel the force of the volleyball hitting my head in high school, moments before I was removed from a gym class for finally losing my shit toward girls who loved to make fun of me because I wasn't a size 2. And there are more memories.

This life of rejection, of disapproval, this is the life I lived for years. It's the life a lot of women—or anyone who doesn't conform to a traditional beauty standard—live. Eventually, these put-downs and the constant barrage of weight-loss ads and marketing tactics by a billion-dollar industry win out. Women cave, spending all of their time, money, and energy on achieving the unattainable beauty standard. How do I know this? Because it is exactly what I did.

After I gave up on athletics, I spent years focused on music and education. I always had a poetic and musical side to me, and because of my body's size, pursuing this nonphysical path just seemed like the right answer, the best option for me to be successful. I even got a fine arts degree and started teaching. But throughout all of that time, I struggled. Even though it had no bearing on my daily tasks, I felt as if nothing I did was ever going to be good enough or appreciated enough until I was living in a thin body. Like many bombarded by diet culture, I assumed that being thin and fit was the key to happiness. That it was the golden ticket to discovering what it's like to achieve your dreams. (Or at least given the permission to reach for them.) I spent years constantly trying to lose weight.

Then everything changed: I had a daughter. After "finally" losing weight, I just gained it right back during my pregnancy. Plus, I suffered from postpartum depression. I lived in a sea of shame and was functioning on an approximate level of WTF. But in moments of clarity, I would remember the most important thing: I had a daughter. All I could think about was that I would *not* let her learn to hate herself the way that I did. And that she would especially not learn any of it from me. I once read a quote from the Instagram account Beauty Redefined that said, "Your body is an instrument, not an ornament,"[1] and it has stuck with me ever since.

So, here I am, keeping that promise to myself. Being true to everything that I know I am. An athlete. A mother. And now, an author. And I have some important things to tell you:

1. Fitness Is for Everybody and Every Body

So, let's get one thing clear right now. Fitness is for everybody and looks different on every body. *No matter* your shape, your size, your background, your capabilities, your strength, or your cardiovascular endurance. (Do you see my point? It bears repeating.) *It's for everybody.* Including the women who have gone most of their lives without ever seeing themselves represented in the fitness world outside of a "before" photo. Including every woman who has ever felt invisible in a world that refuses to see her for more than her body, which is unfortunately, and most likely, every woman.

In the spring of 2015, I was told at my annual gynecologic appointment that I most likely couldn't have a healthy pregnancy because of my weight, because of that specific number penciled on my chart. I was immediately instructed to try dieting and exercise, which was not new advice. But the fear and shame I was filled with pushed me over the edge. So, in full panic mode, I bought some big T-shirts from Walmart, a water bottle, a cheap workout mat, and showed up to a gladiator-style outdoor-group fitness workout. And I threw up everywhere. Literally. I came in dead last on every single exercise we did. I could not transition from the ground to a standing position without pausing to breathe and so missing parts of the workout. I could not move my three-hundred-plus-pound body without feeling as if my bones were about to break. The laughing voices in my head echoed, as years of judgmental eyes and passive-aggressive words regarding my weight flooded my thoughts. I felt helpless. I felt like a body like mine couldn't be called fit—it just wasn't meant for me. I felt like I was constantly some "in-progress" version of me that didn't have the opportunity, much less the permission, to love her body enough to just move for movement's sake. So, I lived with a constant burden. The burden of self-hate. The burden of society's culture screaming at me to change. The burden of giving up and giving in. The burden of being fat.

For years, I spent hours measuring my body, carefully and obsessively weighing it, and exercised solely to lose weight. I did not consider myself someone who is in love with fitness, who thrives off the energy it gives me, who loves gaining muscle, who chugs protein shakes before getting my fitness on, who has competed in powerlifting competitions and combines, and who doesn't give a crap about anyone looking my way as I set up my phone to record myself squatting hundreds of pounds and overhead pressing with sixty-pound dumbbells, and then crushing it because I feel like I crushed it. (Side note: Recording is an incredible way to see how your body moves during a workout. Seeing its *capabilities*, rather than its hindrances, is empowering.)

I believed that narrative handed to me by society. The one screaming "You are not enough" until my ears bled. I envisioned a life for myself that involved symmetrical visible abs and a thigh gap. I craved for the moment my clavicle would finally protrude and be seen. (It never happened, even in the dark pits of my eating disorder.) I would ignore the little moments that were happening. The ones when I completed eight reps instead of five. The times when my squat got a little deeper. The times when I felt faster, my breath less shallow, and my shaking arms seemed just a little less shaky. For years, I ignored the little moments that were slowly but surely changing my life. I pushed them down further and further and pretended that I had no place to own them until my body looked a certain way. So, I looked down more. I squeezed the fat on my sides more. I sucked in more. I stayed in my little corner of the gym more. I didn't feel as if fitness was meant for me. I believed that only a successful weight-loss story would give me the space I didn't even think I deserved to take up.

My mind was filled with so much chaos and negative energy throughout these years. I would search the term *plus-size fitness* and see only exercises being modified for a body like mine. I wanted to grab weights and be a badass, but self-doubt won every single time. I found myself modifying every movement for the entire duration of a workout. I made sure not to push myself too much for fear of hurting myself. I was under the impression that as I was a plus-size woman, things just needed always to be modified. At least until I was no longer the fat girl working out. I was convinced it was going to be impossible for me to dive into fitness until I had a body that looked "fit." I didn't understand that thinness and fitness don't have to be the same thing.

I felt like this until I gave birth to my daughter, Maci. Something clicked as I showed up to work out at eight weeks postpartum. Something inside me screamed as I squatted down, and it brought back memories of feeling as though my bones were about to break again. But something else clicked. I took a deep-ass breath as I shifted my body off my knees into a full plank position. I can still feel the gust of wind that whooshed across my face the moment I began to lower my body downward the best that I could. I got about two inches down and then pushed back up. It was my very first attempt at a push-up that wasn't modified. It wasn't much, but it happened. The feeling of that gust of wind will stay with me forever. It still changes my life every day.

Soon I started sharing these inspirational small moments of mine on social media, and people started paying attention. I get asked "How?" in response to my workouts every single day. There isn't an answer to that question. I complete these workouts because I can, because my body was built for it. I realize this concept is new to a lot of people. It's quite shocking to see a body such as mine do things that "should" be modified. I don't have the traditional "fitness" body. But neither do a lot of the most badass athletes in the world. That's just facts.

So, here's the secret. (But, really, it's no secret. And we'll talk a whole lot more later about why fitness is for every fucking body, among many other things.) Here's a way to give yourself the chance at a gust-of-wind moment:

Know that you are stronger and more capable than you allow yourself to believe. Yes, you! Start with the nonmodified exercise. Even if you can only do one rep, half of one rep, or the tiny beginning of a tiny beginning of the rep, do it. Try it. Sound crazy or impossible? Then you're ready for it.

Promise yourself that you will *always* start without the modification. So what if you finish only one rep? That's still freaking awesome. Just keep at it: transition back to the modification, and on the next set, start with the nonmodified one again. Little by little, my two-inch push-up transitioned into full-range-of-motion push-ups to pauses to balancing on medicine balls all within the last year. I spent my first few years of doing push-ups on my knees, assuming I needed to, assuming that push-ups were meant for a smaller body. The voices in my head and all over the internet shouted that I wasn't ready and that everything needed to be modified for my plus-size body.

Changing the narrative around plus-size bodies and fitness starts by changing the narrative that we tell ourselves. We are capable of doing incredible things with our bodies: it is possible. We are more than just the modification. We are part of the fitness world. Screw the judgments or the looks that may come our way as we step out of our comfort zones. They mean nothing compared to what we can and *will* accomplish when we get out of our own way.

So, show up and get your fitness on. No matter your size or shape.

2. We Are Tired

To be honest, we are so fucking tired.

Tired of sitting at dinner tables filled with anxiety as we consider what others will think of what we eat. Tired of answering questions about our diet habits while waiting to see the doctor for a sprained ankle. Tired of walking into clothing stores and quickly realizing the largest size is seven sizes smaller than what we wear. Tired of watching movies and shows where our bodies are almost never represented or, even when they are, are portrayed as sad or funny—never normal. Tired of all the weight-loss ads promising a new, shinier version by starving ourselves. Tired of being told that losing weight would be the answer to all of our problems. Tired of the fatphobia that sucks the life out of us all and profits off it by the billions. Tired of being called brave for feeling beautiful and sexy in a larger body. Tired of living in a world that celebrates weight loss at literally any cost. It is beyond mentally and emotionally exhausting.

I spent years convinced I wasn't worthy of celebrating my body. I assumed that loving your body was only for those who achieved "better" bodies, smaller bodies. I grew up reading the magazine headlines. I heard the intense screams of Jillian Michaels. I felt the eyes as I stepped into a pool wearing a T-shirt and shorts. I heard the laughs as I drew a heart around my crush's name on my middle school book cover. I felt the shame as the department store worker said, "Sorry, but we don't carry that size." I felt the hunger consume me with every breath. I saw the number on the scale dropping as the number of times I felt self-hate rose. I felt my life passing right by. I believed a truth that was never my own. And I'm still not completely sure how, but somehow, I woke up.

Now I feel hopeful: I know better now, and I refuse to allow this to be my narrative anymore. Now women such as Lizzo are being celebrated. Women such as Tess Holliday are on magazine covers. Now I am celebrating myself, too.

But things don't change overnight. I see the looks of disgust as I begin wearing the clothes that I love. I get criticism for loving fitness but not losing weight. I read comments questioning my health. It still sucks sometimes. And it still hurts. The old narrative still tries to win. But no matter the number of times critics scream "diabetes" or "glorifying obesity," whether it's to make their millions of dollars or whether it's to deal with their own internal battles, I still celebrate.

Society's idea of me is not my narrative anymore. (But I'm exhausted enough by it to last me a lifetime if I choose to let it.)

Because ALL of our bodies are worth the biggest celebration imaginable for being here and our best in a world full of fatphobic, health-concern-trolling bullshit. There, I said it.

We don't need twisted motivational strategies. We need acceptance. We need representation. We need inclusion. We need the message to be that our worth has nothing to do with our weight.

If anyone cares about changing lives, that's the message that will change people. Because for the first time, it will come from a place of self-love, not from a place of self-hate. We are tired of being told to hate ourselves enough to change. We were not born to be forced into miserably shrinking our bodies. We were not born to be labeled. We were not born to be belittled or displaced by society. We were not born to feel like a burden on society.

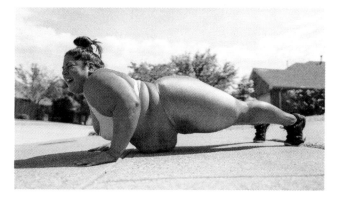

It starts with a simple thank-you. Your body deserves to feel that every once in a while.

We deserve to live out loud and for it to be normal and beautiful to see. To earn promotions. To dance our hearts out. To break records. To lift heavy weights. To fall in love. To wear swimsuits. To be main characters with real and complex story lines. To feel represented. To not hide ourselves anymore. Because shrinking ourselves for the comfort of others has never been the answer. Bodies are meant to be different shapes and sizes. They all deserve to take up the space that they take up. They all deserve respect and love and the opportunity to live a full life.

Now I train several times per week (plus a killer hot yoga sesh). I'm strong as hell—I frequently challenge some of the men that I train with. And I'm the healthiest that I have ever been, both physically and mentally.

For me to begin appreciating my body, I had to let go of this false narrative that the most important aspect of health is what you can see rather than what you can feel. And let me tell you, I *feel* amazing and strong and in love with my journey. (Even though society says I should feel otherwise and that I am not trying hard enough to be thin.)

The way your body looks and is shaped has never been the problem. You owe society nothing. You are allowed to focus on your health without any sort of aesthetic reasoning. Fitness has no size. We've just been conditioned to believe that is does.

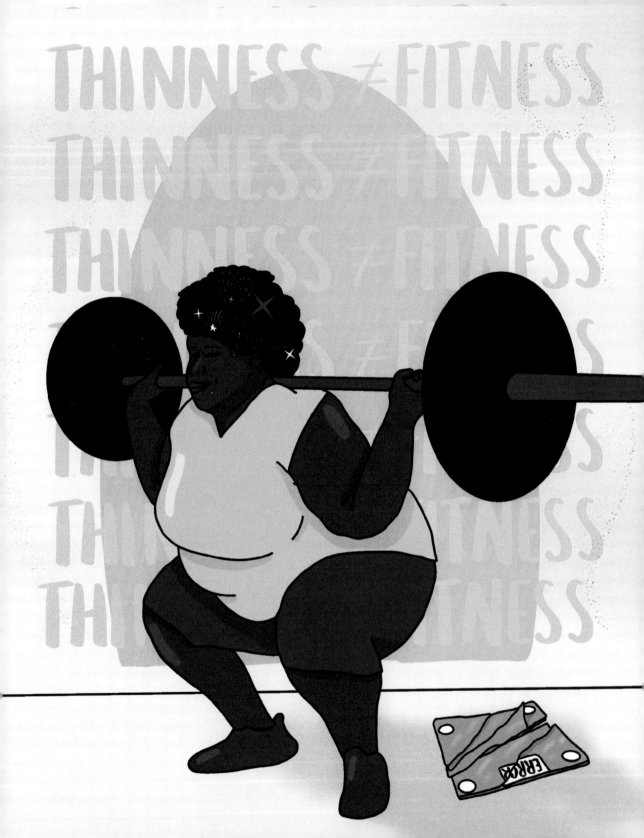

PART 2

The Part Where We Talk about How Thinness and Fitness Are Not the Same Thing

BREAKING UP WITH DIET CULTURE

What Is Diet Culture?

Diet culture might be a new term to you, or it might be a phrase that you've heard over and over as you began unpacking all of the damage it's caused you over your lifetime. Regardless, it's a big part of our society, and a lot of the time we don't even realize its presence until we are trying to escape it, just to find it everywhere we look. Which is fucked-up and infuriating.

So, what exactly is it? Christy Harrison, an anti-diet registered dietitian, nutrition-ist, certified intuitive-eating counselor, and author of *Anti-Diet*, defines diet culture as "a system of beliefs that worships thinness and equates it to health and moral virtue."[2] It encourages weight loss and the pursuit of thinness and societal beauty standards—at all costs. Which usually leaves you with a lifetime of pursuing an impossible thin "ideal" with feelings of failure. Diet culture forces us to become extremely aware of food choices and then filled with shame about meeting one of our most basic human needs. It oppresses bodies that do not meet the "ideal" standards and pictures of "health," which damages the physical and mental well-being of women, those with dis-abilities, people of color, people in larger bodies, and all other marginalized groups. A lot of the negativity that I've experienced as a woman in a larger body throughout my life has stemmed from this culture, which consistently forced me to believe my body was wrong and unworthy.

Diet culture conflates size with health, creating weight stigma.
Diet culture suggests that fat people be stereotyped and shamed and criticized and ha-rassed until they become thin. There is literally a federally funded "war on obesity," which encourages this in the name of "health," sponsored by the US Department of Agriculture obesity-prevention programs. Yet, studies have shown that the failure rate for diets is significantly higher than the success rate of maintaining after weight loss. In November 2018, the NEDA (National Eating Disorders Association) announced new legislation that amends the current USDA obesity-prevention programs to include eating-disorder pre-vention. According to the NEDA, the Long-Term Investment in Education for Wellness (LIVE Well) Act reflects that "weight-inclusive programs that reject an emphasis on weight and weight loss by focusing on health being multifaceted improves the health of individu-als with and without eating disorders."[3] It incorporates eating-disorder prevention within the already existing federal nutrition education (and obesity) programs. So, while there will still be funding for obesity-prevention programs for the foreseeable future, I hope that the LIVE Well Act will provide an opportunity to shift the conversation away from cur-rent weight-focused, fearmongering programs toward weight-inclusive ones that encour-

age overall health and well-being for all sizes, without the weight stigma that continues to negatively affect those labeled as obese. Here are some stats on why changing the conversation is so important:

- There has been a 66 percent increase in weight discrimination over the last decade since the rise of national obesity-prevention campaigns and words such as *BMI* and *obesity epidemic* became part of our national vocabulary.[4]
- Forty to 60 percent of girls aged six through twelve are concerned about their weight or becoming too fat, which endures throughout their lives.[5]
- Of American elementary school girls who read magazines, 69 percent say that the pictures influence their concept of the ideal body shape, and 47 percent say the pictures make them want to lose weight.[6]
- Seventy-nine percent of weight-loss-program participants reported coping with weight stigma by eating more food.[7]
- Ninety-five percent of dieters will regain their lost weight in one to five years.[8]
- A content analysis of weight-loss advertising in 2001 found that more than half of all advertising for weight-loss products made use of false, unsubstantiated claims.[9]
- Americans spend more than $60 billion on dieting and diet products each year.[10]

Diet culture uses movement as a form of punishment.

We become convinced that exercise and movement are specifically for fat prevention and/or fat punishment. (Rather than, oh, I don't know, for fun and enjoyment.) Diet culture also somehow gives others the permission to comment on any sort of movement made in fat bodies with "Good job" and "Way to go" in reference to the assumption that we're exercising specifically to be less fat. (We'll dive much deeper into this in Part 4.)

Diet culture creates thin privilege.

Having thin privilege essentially means that you can enter a restaurant, an airplane, the doctor's office, or any other public place and fit into a seat every single time. There are so many more examples, such as walking into a retail store and being able to try on items. But this isn't something thin people asked for—it was created by a culture that values smaller bodies over all other bodies and only accommodates those that it values. (Nevertheless, thin people should acknowledge that they have this privilege.)

Diet culture is the ultimate gaslighter.

Restrict, punish, restrict, punish, restrict, punish. A lot of the diets we go on (or "lifestyle changes" or whatever euphemism you want to give them) will most likely always feel like famine. Our body's natural instinct is to protect itself—it's why our species has survived for more than 300,000 years—so it'll likely revolt against these changes. Our inner survival instinct is the reason we "hit plateaus" on diets and feel like we completely messed up, which causes us to assume we have these terrible bodies that are undeserving and unworthy and all we have to do is just restrict harder. Punish harder. And so the cycle continues.

Diet culture believes that it's okay to risk the life of a fat person.

It's a do-whatever-it-takes mentality. This tends to lead to eating disorders, disordered eating, broken relationships with food, body dysmorphia, and even, in some cases, death. The same eating disorders being diagnosed in thin bodies are being ascribed to those in fat bodies with active denial of any difference. (Even going so far as to diagnose "atypical" anorexia in fat bodies . . . just because they are fat.) Diet culture prefers fat people to either shrink their bodies into thinness or die trying.

A few years ago, I was willing to die trying. I was willing to believe the lies. I was willing to give up my life in the pursuit of thinness, which I believed would offer happiness. Let me tell you, I lost a ton of weight while starving; while skipping meals for days at a time; while pushing my body out of pure hatred. All this just to find myself in a body almost one hundred pounds less and still considered plus-size. I found myself begging for an escape. Then I discovered two things that helped immensely with breaking the cycle: intuitive eating and body positivity. One of the scariest parts of breaking up with diet culture is figuring out how to heal your relationship with food. The other part is how to handle the emotional toll it takes to see your body changing and possibly gaining weight during recovery.

INTUITIVE EATING

Healing my relationship with food was absolute hell for about a year, if I'm being perfectly honest. I had several moments of wanting to just completely fall back into my old way of trying diet after diet, each one a little more extreme than the last; of spending large chunks of every paycheck on all the shakes and "fat-burning" pills; of skipping meals; of obsessively hanging charts of calorie-exact meals and my weigh-in disappointments all over the fridge. It would take everything in me to stop zooming in on photos of myself while internally pleading for any noticeable change. I was so comfortable in the discomforts of dieting that I had lost sight of any other way of approaching food. (Hello, diet-culture gaslighting curse.)

I was first introduced to the concept of intuitive eating during the pits of my recovery hell. I was feeling triggered by just about everything food-related at the time, so just the word *eating* on yet another "plan" felt almost impossible to even entertain. But within a few weeks, I started reading more on it. Intuitive eating didn't click right away, but I'm not sure where I'd be right now if I hadn't stuck with it.

Registered dietitian Evelyn Tribole is the coauthor of the foremost book on the subject, *Intuitive Eating*, and creator of the ten key principles of intuitive eating, which describes intuitive eating as "a self-care eating framework, which integrates instinct, emotion, and rational thought."[11] There are no guidelines about specific foods to avoid. Instead, intuitive eating focuses on trusting our bodies and their natural intuition.

The Ten Key Principles of Intuitive Eating

1. Reject the diet mentality
2. Honor your hunger
3. Make peace with food
4. Challenge the food police
5. Discover the satisfaction factor
6. Feel your fullness
7. Cope with your emotions with kindness
8. Respect your body
9. Movement—feel the difference
10. Honor your health—gentle nutrition

I know what you're thinking: *Okay, so what does any of this even mean?* I'll break down what I learned from each principle, including a few examples of how I applied it during my eating-disorder recovery while forming a new, healthier relationship with food.

Rejecting the diet mentality almost feels as though you're breaking a law. For me, it felt as if a revolution were erupting from my soul. It's going to most likely feel quite terrifying at first. But the feeling of empowerment that does erupt from taking complete control of your body is exhilarating. It's been a process to digest this revolutionary new way of (literally) surviving as a human being.

To help reject diet mentality, I chose to quit little destructive habits, first hourly, then daily, weekly, and eventually altogether. This meant saying goodbye to:

- Weighing myself (I eventually threw the scale away)
- Tracking my exercises and food intake, either via a chart that I kept on the fridge, or in an app
- Participating in weight-loss discussions

Honor your hunger. Feeling hungry does not mean that your body is failing. There is absolutely nothing to be ashamed about for feeling hungry. It's what our bodies are designed to feel to, you know, stay alive. Somehow, diet culture often has us pairing the sensation of hunger with feelings of shame and guilt. When you think about this logically, and not through the lens of diet culture, it's just absurd.

So to honor my hunger, I started paying attention to:

- The physical sensations in my body when I felt hungry (usually an emptiness, sometimes a growl in my stomach up into my throat)
- How I approached cravings and hunger in terms of my mood (recognizing any internal judgmental thoughts)
- How I felt *after* eating (and how this affected my overall mood)

Make peace with food and give yourself permission to eat. Food is not evil and is certainly not here to ruin your life. We spend so much time being deprived of the foods we love that any chance we get to consume them turns into a moment of guilt and shame. This is pretty crazy, considering we need food to survive. But maybe if we weren't so deprived all the time, we would actually have moments to enjoy fueling our bodies with any of the foods we love.

I started by:

- Introducing previous "forbidden foods" into the house, usually one item at a time. I started with powdered doughnuts. (Yes, it took me a while to find peace with them and not eat most of the bag. This is normal when you first give yourself even the slightest permission. This is not failing.)
- Not immediately shaking my head and looking away when the waiter at a restaurant asks me if I want dessert (and giving myself the chance to ask myself, and I mean ask myself in the most nonjudgmental way, Well, do I?)
- Eliminating the "good" food verses "bad" food values from my vocabulary

Challenge the food police by remembering that eating certain foods does not make you a bad person. This can feel confusing when this idea of judging yourself or another person for eating has so outrageously been normalized by Western society. There is no reason to feel like a terrible person for eating the foods you prefer. This can be an exhausting principle because the food police lives and breathes within us every moment of every day. Even when we're no longer physically tracking every calorie, our minds might keep adding it all up.

The moments when I start feeling judgmental toward myself for what I eat, I ask myself:

- Why is this a food rule for me? (For me, I mostly found that it always led me back to the attachment of the phrase "it makes you fat.")
- Why do I give this food any moral value?
- Do I actually feel bad about this food or do I feel upset about what the food "potentially does" to my body, which might in turn change people's perspective on how I'm treated and respected as a human being?

Discover the satisfaction factor and eat what you actually want to eat. As soon as I adopted the practice of intuitive eating, I realized right away that diet culture had stripped away my connection to my personal food preferences. I wasn't even sure what I liked because I had only ever known the difference between "good" and "bad" foods, forcing me to lose sight of which foods I loved as opposed to foods that I only craved due to restriction.

I started eating foods again to simply eat, choosing ones I thought I might like. I also:

- Asked myself, Do I like spicy foods? (I had no idea that I did not like spicy food until I gave myself permission to eat it whenever I want.)
- Made sure that I knew the answer to What am I *actually* craving right now?
- Made a list of foods that I simply liked. (I eventually learned that I love flavorful salads, but only enjoy them when I *want* to eat them.)

Feel your fullness by paying attention to signs from your body that let you know that you are full. And not the kind of full where you're feeling sick and incredibly uncomfortable. (I believe that this is a common misconception about intuitive eating and the anti-diet movement when referring to "feeling full.") Listen to your body and trust it.

I started paying attention to what I was doing while I was eating:

- Noticing if I was distracted by watching TV, having conversations, or just plain doing other things while I ate
- Using my left hand to eat (I'm a righty) to help myself pay attention a little more to the actual eating and tasting of my food
- Taking intentional breaks to tune in to what the food tasted like, what the texture felt like, and allowing myself to taste that bite during my intentional pause

Cope with your emotions with kindness because food does not magically resolve our internal emotional discomfort. Now, food might numb it for a few minutes or hours. Food might create a distraction for us to focus on instead of facing the struggles we face emotionally. But when the dust settles and the numbing fades, we are right back to where we started: face-to-face with the source of our discomfort. And it can quickly become an obsessive and unfortunate cycle. One we truly don't deserve.

When I feel myself heading toward using food as a distraction from something I'm not ready to face:

- I ask myself, How am I feeling in this very moment?
- I draw a circle chart and color in the emotions I am feeling
- I ask myself, What could I use right now to help? (I've found myself realizing I needed rest, or a hug, or just some quiet time for myself.)

Respect your body and its shape and size. We aren't genetically made to all look exactly the same. Some of us have larger feet and smaller hands. Some of us are tall and some of us are short. Some of us have square butts and some of us have round butts. That's just basic human DNA. And even with that, it's okay for your body to change and evolve over time. Because, news flash, all bodies are damn good ones. No matter how they look.

The first steps I took were to:

- Look in the mirror at least once a day for more than a minute at a time
- Unfollow all accounts on social media that made me feel like shit about myself (while following those that make me feel respected and accepted as I am)
- Wear clothes that feel comfortable (I ended up bagging up and donating clothes that I was still trying to squeeze into because I refused to buy the next size up)

Feel the difference when you move your body. Rather than focus on the number of calories you need to burn to make up for the food you ate, allow yourself to feel the sensation of movement and notice how these sensations make you feel. Movement is a primal instinct. Maybe we enjoy the quick bursts of movement and maybe that brings us the most joy. Or maybe picking up a ton of weights brings us the most joy. Whatever kind of movement is providing that for us, the last thing it should bring us is shame and punishment.

I began to ask myself:

- What activities have I enjoyed in my lifetime? (Strength based were always at the top of my list, but cardio had always been advised for me since it "burns fat" more than any other exercise.)
- What did I enjoy about them? (I loved how empowered they made me feel. Turned out I was craving that feeling in all my activities.)
- Are there other pastimes that are similar to what I enjoy that I haven't tried yet? (This is how I found my passion for powerlifting.)

Honor your health with gentle nutrition and choose foods that make you feel physically well. I used to be willing to suffer from excruciating stomachaches after eating fried onion rings because I would become obsessed with eating foods that I hadn't previously allowed myself. (Ugh, I swear if I had a nickel for every food I've shoved down my throat just in spite of its being restricted and then finding myself regretting it due to internal repercussions—yeah, I'd be rich.) And, you know what? I don't even like onions.

I started asking myself:

- If it's making me feel so terrible physically, do I really like the food? Enough to be this miserable? (Definitely going to be a no from me.)
- Are there foods that make me feel the opposite? Strong and fulfilled? (Yup—come at me, steak and potatoes.)
- Which foods offer me both physical fulfillment *and* make my taste buds smile? (My list has slowly grown as I began differentiating between what I liked and what I was scared I'd never get to have again.)

For a full list of resources and to learn more about Intuitive Eating, please turn to page 191.

• • •

We are craving these positive, open conversations more and more. We want to feel confident in our bodies; to feel at home in them; to love the parts of us we can see and touch and attempt to embrace. We call these desires many things: body confidence; body acceptance; body neutrality. We read the self-help books. Recite positive quotes. Create Pinterest boards as reminders.

But there's a part of acceptance that can be hard to sit with. We forget to ask or avoid altogether asking ourselves, Why? Why do we even need these new layers? How did we even become so wounded with these negative body-image thoughts? What is it we are so afraid of?

In looking for these answers, we often avoid any of the reasons. We avoid any of the deepest, darkest truths. We avoid admitting that we are terrified of appearing or becoming fat. We avoid our fatphobia. It's not our fault. And it's okay to admit it. It's okay to peel back broken layers first. It's okay if we have to start small. It's okay to be scared when it gets uncomfortable, when we realize we can't change overnight, when we just need a moment to sit with that for a while. I had to just sit with it for a good while, too.

I Was Enough

The goal was never to find myself.

Or change. Or become who I'm meant to be.

I was just afraid.

Terrified, quite frankly.

Of actually allowing myself to just be me.

I knew who I was. Deep down, at least.

She was there all this time.

And she worried me.

She didn't quite fit in.

I thought I needed to change her into something
a little bit better. A little less potty-mouthed.
A little more beautiful. A little less round
shaped. A little more soft-spoken.

I thought maybe that was the key.

I thought maybe that was healing.

I thought maybe that was growth.

And yet, it was all far from it.

Finding myself was never the goal.

Being myself was enough.

All this time, I was enough.

FITNESS DOES *NOT* REQUIRE THINNESS

I once passed a billboard that said in giant, bold letters LOSE WEIGHT. FINALLY, LIVE HAPPY AND HEALTHY. This message is not only old and outdated, it's dangerous. The association made between weight loss and happiness mixed with this false sense of "finally" achieving the dream life is killing people. Yet it's still everywhere.

We live in a world where appearance is one of the most important factors for success in life, especially for women. Women are judged for not wanting to lose weight and for wanting to lose weight. For wearing too much makeup, for not wearing enough. For dressing too sexy, for dressing too casually. For getting Botox, for not shaving, for keeping bushy eyebrows, for having our panty lines showing, for getting hair and lash extensions, for posting photos of our cellulite and stretch marks, for being too modest, for being too sexy. I mean, for fuck's sake. Women are tired of this narrative that only one body type is acceptable. Women's bodies are damn miracles. And we get to decide what we do or don't do with them. Every body is different. And different is *not* wrong.

So what if my stomach hangs? Especially when I do push-ups. I'm a fitness beast.

I have all of these marks and rolls. So what? I am more than the weight or shape or size or color or softness of my body. And so are you. When I was first seen moving my body, exercising, and following all the fat girl weight-loss trends, it was applauded while being seen as both expected and necessary. And when I slapped on a crop top in the gym, whoa. Listen to the crowds roar. Suddenly, I was *brave*.

It took a while for me to realize how hard it was on my soul to hear myself being called brave repeatedly just for being happy in my body. At first, it felt good. Like, *Wow, hell yeah, I'm brave.* Eventually, it still kind of felt good, but it sort of felt odd. I got to a place where I actually had moments of being unconcerned about my body rolls and marks and bumps. I was laughing and soaking in actual life moments. I was wearing what felt comfortable in hot weather. I was working out without the intention of getting smaller.

Suddenly, I was brave for doing these things and posting about them. It felt confusing for me. I was so brave for allowing myself to be seen? No, it was implied that it's brave to do that knowing I will be judged and shamed for just being me. Understanding that became hard. The bravery comments turned into an unfortunate insult, even from the kindest people who had no ill intentions. At least that's how it all began to feel.

But this is not bravery. This is just how my body folds. It's just the position it takes when I sit or when I squat three hundred pounds for fun. And it makes lots of other shapes as well when I move.

This is my home.

I took my first breaths in this body, this home. I learned to walk and run in this home. I discovered my voice in this home. I played musical instruments in this home. I created life in this home. I became an athlete in this home. I found love for this home. We all have a home we've lived in since birth. It's not brave for showing it some love. It's just part of the incredible journey we all go on when we get the opportunity to furnish one with a whole lot of love, a bunch of appreciation, and more memories than we can count.

YOU ARE NOT A "BEFORE"

I used to consider myself a "before," falsely believing that my body was only temporary. This lie is what made me feel accepted. It's what allowed me to feel as though there was space for me. I was a "Don't worry, I'm going to change this" while internally screaming I was a "Yes, I know, I'm working on it," while hoping the conversation would end. I was a "Yes, this is temporary, I'm going to look better" while exhaling a soft sigh through glazed-over eyes. All these befores made me feel like garbage—even as the befores began to transition into my hopeful "after," that after still always felt like a before. Because I was always going to be a before, someone that desperately needed to be changed. I had stopped living a real life.

But I slowly started to let go of that. I started to have little moments of accidental togetherness with myself. I'd see the squishy parts of me that shake when I laugh. I'd see the crazy-in-love look on my husband's face as his hand grazed my side right before we closed our eyes to sleep. I'd notice how the chills it gave me came from love, not embarrassment. I'd feel my stomach touch the ground when my arm strength had built up enough to do regular push-ups on my toes. I'd notice how it's possible to be strong at any size. I'd glance at my smile as I passed mirrors. And realize that I'd noticed something other than the size of my waist or the jiggle in my thighs. I'd notice all of these tiny moments of just simply living as I am. Living in *my* body, just the way that it is. And it is not, and has never been, just a before.

During the years I spent focused on losing weight, I lived for the comments surrounding my body and its "progress" toward becoming the "after" photo. I couldn't ever get enough of hearing:

"Wow! You look amazing!"

"Such an inspiration!"

"I barely even recognize you!"

"How did you do it?!"

It was like a rush of dopamine every time that I heard something like this. It was my validation that I had worth. But I don't need it anymore. I'm so much more athletic than I was when I craved those words. I'm stronger. I'm faster. I'm healthier. I'm happier. I'm actually living. For a lot of people, that's a little less exciting to notice because it's not the change that we have been conditioned to praise. In my life now, there are no more "I'm dying to know how you did it" conversations. No more "You look amazing" confirmations. Until I let go of them, I hadn't realized that they weren't ever helping me, only hurting me. And you know what? Not hearing them now, I feel more worthwhile than ever before.

We can't hate ourselves into change—which is exactly what we're trying to do when we focus on the "before." But we sure as hell can pride ourselves into growth, into getting uncomfortable, into discovering our truth, into creating a space in our hearts for self-love. So have pride. Even if you have to take a break. Even if you have to cry it out because it just feels that good and difficult and real and possible. Feeling proud doesn't come after you reach the destination. Feeling proud happens when you open your heart to the possibility of applauding the step you're on today. Allow yourself to focus on your health without trying to shrink your body. To weigh yourself in your kindness, in your creativity, in your strengths, in the difference you make for those around you, in the ways that feel authentic to you. Because, to me, that's what matters. Not some number on a scale. For me, I find my worth in my laughter. I find it in my sweaty grunts during lifts. I find it in all of the little moments where I'm living and breathing and loving it all. This body, on this day, however we are.

* * *

I once heard a piece of self-help advice that has stuck with me: to build confidence, you should say something like "Dang, I'm the bomb" in the mirror. Even if you don't feel like it, you should try to say it as if you mean it. This seemed weird to me because, at the time, I wasn't remotely close to feeling like "the bomb." So, yeah, it didn't work every time, at least not right away. But I will never forget the first time I tried it. I was in a decent mood, so I gave it a shot. I felt so silly that it made me laugh out loud. Maybe it was just the nervous energy, but it felt kind of good, even if it didn't convince me in that moment.

We've been so conditioned to put ourselves down through years of the diet-culture mind-set that even praising ourselves while we are alone simply looking in a mirror feels silly. We constantly brush off any compliments given to us and completely downplay our accomplishments. Maybe we have this fear of being perceived as full of ourselves or conceited. Maybe we have just been told *so many times* that the flesh and bones that make up our bodies could look *so much better*. Maybe we've been told that our strengths are only strengths if matched with unattainable beauty. Maybe we feel that we need to be in the gym as often as humanly possible to ensure we reach a level of thinness that would render us beautiful. Well, you know what? Fuck that.

We are allowed to love whatever the hell we want about ourselves. We can be proud of who we are. We can do whatever makes us feel at home, happy, and free of the pressure. It is my hope that we all just try to start saying, "I'm the bomb." (Like you mean it. Because there's a good chance that one day you will.) It's okay if you get frustrated on this path toward body acceptance/confidence/neutrality. (You will get frustrated.) You will have some bad days. You will catch yourself comparing yourself to other people. It might make you angry that you might never be accepted. This will all be extremely frustrating. It will seem impossible. You will feel as if it's no longer worth trying.

But here's the truth:

None of us are confident every second. Not even me. I have days when I have such a difficult time just looking in the mirror. It can feel suffocating to realize your internalized fatphobia is sneaking out. It gets confusing and messy a lot of the time. And I still catch myself analyzing my stomach folds before I post to Instagram. I still catch myself thinking twice, feeling as though I might be taking up too much space.

We all have terrible, straight-up shitty days. This journey to self-love is hard. And comparing ourselves to other people just makes it even harder. It helps to remember that we are all trying our best through the frustrations and roadblocks. I know that a lot of us want to cancel our internal fatphobic thoughts. I know I do. Some days are just a lot more difficult than others.

I used to fantasize about what it might be like to wake up one day and look physically different. Would I feel happiness for the first time? I would imagine myself walking into rooms and being noticed, being given incredible opportunities. I found myself thinking of all the clothes that I would wear in this new life. Would I take more selfies? Would I be more outspoken? Years went by, and I still woke up the same. The fantasy would never come true, even after all the dieting and overexercising. I eventually had to realize that what I was wanting was far from what I thought was the truth. So, I took a chance, even though it felt scary. I started taking selfies and trying out new hairstyles. I wore the clothes that I liked (because it turned out I had a style). I started speaking my truths—all without my fantasy ever happening. And that's when I saw what my fantasy was really about: I wanted to live in a world where regardless of what I looked like, I'd still receive respect and be given equal opportunities. It turns out that I could get that respect by being confident in myself.

I know that this is hard to do, though. It's going to get frustrating. But that's okay. You're not doing a bad job of loving yourself and feeling confident. These frustrations are normal. Keep going. Because here I am. And here we all are. Taking up our fucking space. With open arms for all else who are ready to take up theirs as well. This is how revolutions begin.

Say This, Not That

Here are a few suggestions on how to redirect those toxic internal thoughts (and sometimes external comments) that might creep back up when you're on a journey toward self-confidence and self-acceptance.

"I feel fat."

- What are you really feeling? Tired, lazy, gross? (Because fat is not a feeling.) By using *fat* to describe these other states of being, you're implying that to be fat is to be inherently lazy and gross. When I hear this, I remember that diet culture loves to remind me that my body is gross and bad at any weight that includes body fat. Which isn't true; weight gain is normal. Bodies change sometimes.

- Instead, try saying, "I'm not feeling very good about my body today." (Because even if you *are* fat, it does not mean that your body is bad, wrong, or gross.)

"Does this make me look fat?"

- Would that be a bad thing? Are you afraid to look fat? By asking yourself this, you're implying that anyone who is fat looks bad. Looking or being fat doesn't immediately mean you look bad. (If an article of clothing makes you feel good and is comfortable on your body, I'm guessing you look amazing.)
- Instead, try, "What do you think of this outfit?"

"You're not fat, you're beautiful."

- First of all, I'm both. (Because, yes, that's possible.)
- Instead, try the simple, "You're beautiful."

"Don't call yourself fat!"

- Are you seeing the trend here? Fat is not an insult. It's simply a description.
- Instead, try nothing. People should be allowed to describe themselves however they choose to. (Yet, if it's people who are clearly thin, maybe ask them what emotion they are really feeling. And remind them that fat is not a feeling.)

"I need to lose like ten pounds."

- Do you *really need* to lose ten pounds? Almost certainly not.
- Instead, try, "I would love to explore a healthier relationship with my body."

For a full list of body image resources, please turn to page 194.

Being Her

Parts of her were gone.

Missing pieces she thought she might not ever see
again.

The parts that were endlessly scraped away from
her the moment she began to understand.

The moment she began to see the laughter.

The pointing fingers.

The words left in her in-box.

The denial to live as she was.

So many parts of her felt dead.

Only pieces of her left on the floor.

She was changed.

But on a random Thursday, with what felt like weak
hands,

She picked up one of the pieces.

And felt her entire body begin to shake.

Begin to move.

Begin to burn bright.

Before she knew it, she fell down to her knees.

And began to scrape up every piece she could find.

She heard laughter nearby as she scooped up piece after piece.

But she didn't care this time.

This time, she chose herself.

For the first time, she felt what it was like to be whole.

To actually be her.

AN OPEN LETTER
TO THE FITNESS INDUSTRY

A lot of us fold in places we are told we shouldn't fold. We might dimple in places we are told we should keep covered. When I'm vocal about this, I'm told that I'm just glorifying obesity. But I'm done being apologetic about it. I'm done apologizing for existing and loving fitness in my fat body. I'm done tiptoeing around real issues that real women are facing. The women who post their untouched photos and receive criticism. The women with bruised hips from a salon chair that they didn't quite fit in. The women who smile with excitement when the words *size inclusive* and *body positive* are included on a brand's website, only to realize that the extended sizing still ends four sizes below theirs. The women avoiding doctors for fear of not being believed for the hundredth time. The women afraid of entering a gym without being criticized for not choosing the ultimate weight-loss plan. The women who have never seen their body type on a mannequin in activewear before.

Some of these women are hiding from a world that they are constantly excluded from, and it is hurting their mental health. Some of these women are exhausted by stereotypical #fitspo marketing and advertisements when all they want to do is enjoy moving their bodies.

It's hard enough for women to embrace their real bodies in a world full of Photoshop and face-distortion apps. It's that much harder when you as an industry exclude us in every fitness space, whether intentionally or not. Including the trans women and trans men who would love to for once feel seen and acknowledged. And the folks with disabilities who have been waiting for far too long for accessible options.

I work out without any weight-loss goals. I could not care less if working out the way I do results in weight loss. Maybe it will at times and maybe it won't. Either way, I'm proud of my body. And I will continue to thank it every day. For some reason, this seems to come off to some as a radical concept. But it's not. It's opening the door for all people to know that they can step foot into a gym without feeling as if they can only continue showing up if their bodies are continuously shrinking and conforming to a fitness ideal.

Health doesn't always look like a size 2 or 6 or 10 or whatever is currently socially acceptable. It doesn't always look like the least amount of fat possible on someone's body.

A lot of the time, health looks like anyone at any size continuing to show up for themselves in whatever ways feel best for their bodies.

We all fold and bend and roll in places we're told that we shouldn't. Our real bodies are fascinating. Beautiful and ever changing. They are deserving of respect. They are also deserving of clothes, chairs, medical care, and basic human rights.

So, please. Include us. *All* of us. People of *every* size, shape, and color. Trans women of every size, shape, and color. Nonbinary athletes. LGBTQ athletes. Disabled athletes. *All* athletes. Create inclusive fitness spaces that are accessible and filled with respect toward all bodies. Allow us to *finally* be seen. Because the more of us that begin to feel represented and acknowledged and *worthy*, the more of us will give ourselves the chance to realize our own potential. Because, for the first time, we might be able to open a fitness app and see someone who has a body type similar to ours kicking ass (in badass activewear that comes in our size!). Because, for the first time, we'll walk into a gym and see images that represent and celebrate our bodies in their current moment (not just as a before or an after). Because we'll (probably for the first time ever) look in the damn mirror and say, "I'm an athlete" . . . and mean it.

I think we can agree that we all would love for our world to be healthier. Right? So start including us, start seeing us as human beings, as capable athletes of every size. Not just as "before" photos and potential weight-loss journeys to market to the masses. We don't accept that anymore. Because we are athletes. (Oh, and just FYI—we're extremely badass.)

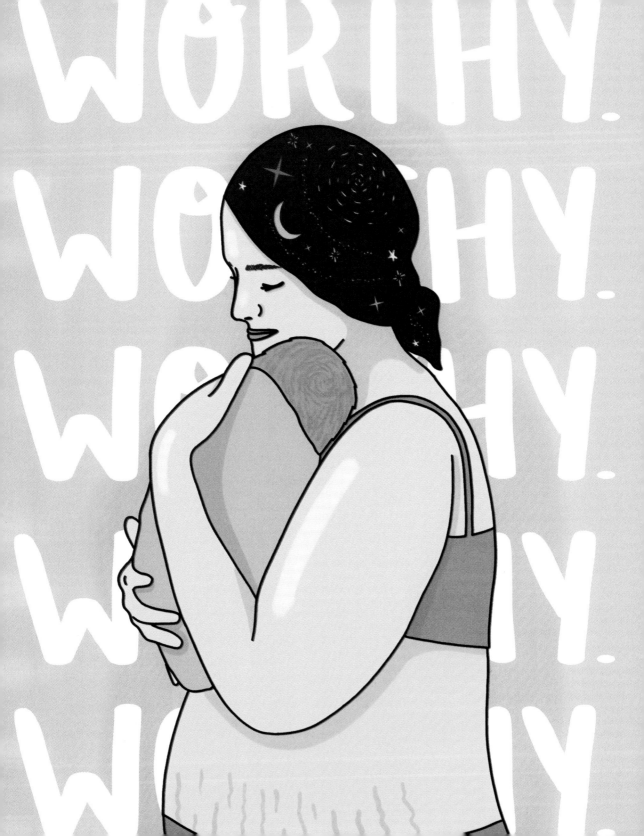

PART 3

The Part Where We Give Moms a Freakin' Break

FIRST OF ALL, MOMS ARE WARRIORS

Maybe you're a mom. Maybe you're a soon-to-be mom. Maybe you're a hopeful mom. Maybe you're none of the above. But if you're a woman, or if one happened to give birth to you, a fair warning that this is about to get fucking real. Because it's time for an honest conversation about how postpartum women are consistently reminded by the fitness industry that they need to "bounce back" during one of the most fragile and overwhelming times in their lives. (Which also is one of the most empowering and straight-up badass times in a woman's life, too.) Yet, postpartum women often spend this time feeling invisible and broken, as they are constantly bombarded by pressures to not only be perceived as, but also to physically look like, the world's perfect mom.

I See You, Mama

I see you, mama. Looking in the mirror picking at everything you see.

I see you, mama. Wondering why you don't look like the other women on your Instagram feed.

I see you, mama. Assuming you aren't worthy enough to post that photo showing off your curves.

I see you, mama. Giving in to temptation because you think it's what your body deserves.

I see you, mama. Forgetting how beautiful you truly are in every single way.

I see you, mama. Crying in the shower almost every single day.

I see you, mama. Afraid of comments that could potentially be hateful.

I see you, mama. Holding in your feelings about your body because someone might tell you that you're ungrateful.

I see you, mama.

This is your reminder for today. . . . You are a warrior, in every single way.

In my experience, most of the clichés about motherhood turned out to be true. When you meet your baby, you burst at the seams with a love that is deeper than any other you've ever known. You cry from happiness and complete fear at the exact same time. There is nothing you wouldn't do for babies to make their lives full of hope, meaning, and love. Looking back, I'm not even sure what I expected when I became a mother on November 4, 2017. I hadn't read any books on expecting a child or impending parenthood, but I'm not sure they would have helped. So, I didn't have this great master plan on the kind of mother I would be.

When I announced my pregnancy, it opened a floodgate of questions and opinions. Do you plan on breastfeeding? Will you homeschool? Are you choosing organic products? What is your goal weight? The queries and comments felt never-ending. And I didn't ever have any of the answers. (Well, except goal weight. I feel that every woman feels as though she has to have a goal weight at all times. Seriously, diet culture is the fucking worst.) I had just one goal in mind: to give my daughter the best life that I could possibly give, whatever that looked like and however that changed as she grew into the person she would eventually become. Even with that singular goal in mind, it was overwhelming to navigate this need to prove that I was a good mom, that I was doing everything "right," and that I was working on getting the "pre-baby body back." I was plagued by constant self-doubt.

But I discovered a little secret, one that is frowned upon by the social media critics and the countless ads screaming that *you are not good enough.* I learned that what is "right" for me is going to sometimes look different from other people's "right" for them. I began noticing other moms sharing their real and raw motherhood truths on Instagram, and little by little I was feeling less and less alone. I wasn't the only one with a messy house and a devastating breastfeeding journey. I wasn't the only one feeling the pressure of "losing the baby weight" and being fully engulfed by mom guilt, shame, and fears. I was turning to social media more and more for a sense of community and relatability. For those moments to remind me that I'm doing the best I can. And you know what? I still doubt myself a lot as a mother all the time and I probably will for the rest of my life. This roller coaster of emotions that comes with motherhood is nothing to be ashamed of. Because every mother trying her best is an amazing parent.

These doubting moments also usually happen when loads of laundry are waiting to be folded on the couch. Or when the microwave won't stop beeping to alert you that your leftover lunch is ready, a meal you've already heated up three times today. Or when you sit and breathe long enough to see the mess that is your house. Or when you see your hairy legs and unwashed hair from the mirror across the room, immediately regretting having skipped your workout this morning. Or when you see the dog bones, two empty water bottles, and an inch of banana under the couch as you sit on your living room floor, exhausted because you feel like you're doing this all wrong. Or when you internally make a list of everything you should be doing right now. Your mind begins to race about everything that needs to get done. And just as you are about to get up, you glance down and see love.

And you're reminded that what you need to be doing is right here in front of you, among the mess, and the beeping, and all of the background noise; you're reminded that you're doing it just right.

I start all of my days with crusty eyes and next-level dragon breath. Then I wash up. Make the bed. Start a load of laundry. Make breakfast in my undies. Sip coffee as Maci runs circles around the island and between my legs. Brush her hair. Serve breakfast. Get her dressed. Prepare my workout drinks. Pack her bag. Put on my workout clothes. And finally sit back down to read her some books before we head out the door to the gym. Before the next wave of the day—the post–9:00 a.m. wave—washes in. It's a lot, and I, like every mom, do my best. The last thing moms need added to that to-do list is a "bounce back" checklist that has nothing to do with being a great mom and more times than not steals away some of the most beautiful parts about motherhood.

There was a lot that I just didn't know when I first became a mom. Like how much I would cry. Or the amount of poop that I would get under my nails. Or how much I'd snort, laugh, and cry at the same time on my kitchen floor in moments of defeat. Or what it would feel like when I'd hear her belly laugh for the first time. Or how much I would cry in the mirror, wishing to look like anyone else but me. I didn't know that everything would feel confusing. Or that I'd have moments I would honestly want it to just all go away. I was unaware I'd be brimming with guilt and fulfillment all at once.

I soon realized that I needed to let my guilt go. Postpartum bodies don't just "bounce back" to normal. (As if "normal" were a thing.) I remembered that my body did something quite magical. It made space to create a life. Remembering this picked me back up from those cries on the kitchen floor. I scooped Maci up and gave her kisses and caused those first belly laughs. It kept me going even when I didn't believe that my body could. And if that's not the definition of a warrior body, then I don't know what is.

I was told a few things about postpartum here and there during my pregnancy. These were usually passing comments like "Stock up on pads" and "Take your time when you go to the bathroom afterwards" and things like that. There was never much detail provided. I never heard anyone's "postpartum story," unless it was referencing plans to fix the problems of a postpartum body. But from the moment Maci was out, shit pretty much hit the fan with the arrival of a vaginal explosion, constipation station, sleep deprivation, pee city nation, and an anxiety-filled depression that would send me straight near the edge of my sanity. And, yes, looking back at it now, I can see why you don't want to scare an already-scared pregnant woman (or give a superhappy pregnant woman a total buzzkill). However, for me, it might have helped to know the feeling of complete brokenness will not last forever. Or that one of the brightest moments of my life could potentially be met with some of the deepest and darkest. It would have helped to know that it's possible for everything to be okay. And that it's okay to talk about it. Postpartum can feel like this constant, delicate dance on the edges of both fear and joy. And for new moms, it often feels as if the joy edges are the only options for us to express our individual experiences without the judgment and shame.

On the day I came home from the hospital with newborn Maci, I was swollen, and everything felt out of place. I thought my body would never again be the same. I feared that all the "work" I had put into becoming strong and healthy (my definition of this at the time) had officially disappeared forever. I walked slowly and couldn't even think about exercising. It seemed impossible. But four weeks later, I tried. I attempted to move my body however it could move. Another month later, I kept trying. I moved my feet fast enough to consider it a jog. I lifted a light dumbbell the best that I could. Another two months later, I packed some weight on my shoulders and did barbell squats. I grabbed a heavier set of dumbbells anytime I could. By the summer of 2018, I was adding more and more weight to the bar. I was passing personal records from my thinner pre-pregnancy days. I was changing, that's for sure, but the mirror wasn't. What I saw in my reflection wasn't looking any different from on the day I looked at my postpartum self in the hospital bathroom mirror. My stomach still hung down low, and that frustrated me. The scale said the same thing as before. My jean size wasn't any smaller than it was before. I had a choice to make and it was terrifying. I could give up and cave into self-hate. Or I could add more weight to the bar, get up off my knees when I did push-

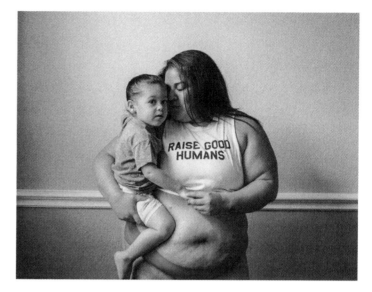

Every month, I make an effort to snap a photo with Maci to replace my once-monthly progress photos with photos of vulnerability embracing the home she first grew in.

ups, and enjoy how it felt when I would beat my personal records. Before motherhood, I would never even have considered anything other than punishing myself for "not working hard enough."

But I now I had someone else to inspire. This time, Maci would be watching. And maybe she wouldn't notice right away, but over time, she would see the way I treated myself, and she would likely treat herself the same. That realization hit me harder than any other had ever hit me in my entire life. So, while it was hard and went against just about everything I had previously believed about fitness and fulfillment, my perspective began to shift.

This Is Postpartum

It wasn't the story I had hoped to share.

Not a journey that seemed all that fair.

It wasn't the goddess-like vision I assumed was
   for me.

Not the moments I ever thought I would see.

But it was still magic and madness and so full of
   love.

It had ups and downs and all of the above.

It gave me strength and power to understand how
   to heal.

It allowed me to learn grace through every
   emotion I would feel.

And even though I sometimes wish my journey had changed its direction.

The universe knew what it was doing when it made its selection.

I found myself through my postpartum journey in so many ways.

I also found out "bounce back" is just bullshit rhetoric from old, stigmatized days.

I let go of the "get skinny at all costs" mentality and focused on fitness as an exercise in fulfillment. It didn't all happen right away. But it was happening bit by bit because I recognized that I was strong and capable no matter what my body physically looked like. Because it was the movement and feeling alive that made me feel good and was helping my postpartum body begin to heal and build strength.

There is no definition of what a postpartum body is supposed to look like, contrary to the messages in ads that target postpartum women. Some women have no marks; some have many. Some women have stomachs that went right back to being smooth and flat; some have a stomach that hangs with loose skin. Some women have lots of fat on their bellies; some have close to none. Some women were following a fitness routine when they got pregnant; some hadn't worked out since grade school when they got pregnant. Some women continued their fitness routine throughout most of their pregnancy, while others kept it at a minimum, and both of these groups of women may have gained extra weight. But they all have a postpartum body worth being proud of. They have a story that counts.

When I first thought about openly sharing my postpartum journey through an online platform, I hesitated. It was such a vulnerable time in my life. I constantly questioned myself, thinking maybe I was sharing too much. I wondered if what I had to say mattered. I wondered if my weirdness was showing too much, if my belly rolls were showing too much, if my insecurities were showing too much. I wondered if I looked too happy on days that I just wasn't. And usually, in each moment of hesitation, I ended up working my way through some sort of positive self-talk (even if it didn't feel like truths in the moment) to remind myself that my story matters. My breastfeeding story, my postpartum story, my birth story, my fitness story, my self-love story, my motherhood story, my life story—they all matter, even if they aren't perfect or what we perceive as "the norm." Because maybe, just maybe, one person might read it or see it and have the feeling for the first time of not being alone.

I was twelve weeks postpartum when I grabbed a pair of scissors and turned one of my shirts into a crop top. As I stood in front of the camera, my hands were trembling. I was about to take a full-body photo of myself for the first time in what felt like forever. Fear took over my body and I immediately closed my eyes. I tried for a smile as I heard the camera shutter click. Even though my heart was racing, I was focused on avoiding my natural instinct to suck it all in. Little did I know that this moment, this decision, would be incredibly pivotal on my journey toward where I am now. This would be the first of many photos I would take. These were photos for which I'd eventually have the courage to reveal my entire belly, to have a real smile for a smile. These were photos where I'd look directly at the camera and finally believe in my worth.

But despite the steps I was taking toward self-love, I felt very alone in what I was sharing as a plus-size mother. Everywhere I looked on Instagram, no new mothers looked like me. So even though I knew there would be criticism, I believed it was important for me, and for others like me, to share my story. And to post the photos and talk about it. Because this is postpartum. No one's is exactly the same as another's.

During the of summer 2018, I began reaching out to mothers I had connected with on Instagram and asked if they would be interested in sharing their postpartum experiences with me on their social media platforms through a project called #this_is_postpartum. The mission was to help mothers understand that they are not alone in their experiences and struggles with embracing their postpartum bodies in whatever shape, size, or form they come. I hoped to represent as many postpartum experiences as possible. By that September, with shaky hands, twenty incredible women hit "post" at the same time and shared their postpartum stories with the world. I never expected the response to create waves the way that it did. But by May 2019, when I recruited another twenty-five women to join hands again, there were thousands of responses online. All celebrating our similarities, our differences, and all of the little things in between that make each of us so incredibly unique. Women have continued to share their stories using the hashtag, and it has grown steadily over the years.

Here are just a few of their powerful stories:

What I really wish I'd known is that all of these feelings of unworthiness, self-hatred, and the deep desire to change what my body looked like were rooted in a false ideal created by the patriarchy. I'm angry. Angry that I grew up wishing, even praying, for my body to be smaller. I thought that maybe if my stomach would flatten out, or if my legs would tone up, or if I could just erase the bloodred stretch marks that spread on my arms and thighs by age thirteen . . . that maybe, just maybe people would like me. Maybe I'd finally have true friendships. Maybe I'd finally have the confidence to do things I loved like sing, act, dance, and play basketball.

Maybe I'd stop trying to hide myself and constantly make myself smaller.

But no matter what I did, how small I forced my body to be, it was never enough. It never took that pain away. It never filled the void of feeling like I wasn't enough.

I spent my college years and entire twenties continuing to try and shrink myself while searching for external validation from everyone I came into contact with. I began exercising, which turned into an unhealthy obsession.

Fast-forward to now. . . . I'm five years postpartum with two daughters and I refuse to let history repeat itself. I'm still angry. I watch countless women let diet culture continue to destroy their lives. It's like a plague. But I won't ever stop fighting for myself, for you, for our children. So that maybe they have a chance at living a good, authentic life based on self-trust and self-respect.

—Ashley Dorough,
houseofdorough.com
(@ashley_dorough)

I have never felt more alone than I have after giving birth. As a Black woman, we're seen as these pillars of strength that overcome everything. And we do. But it's hard. I was a single mom when I birthed my oldest, Kalima. I didn't know what to expect. After she was born, I had one visitor in the hospital outside of my mom. Goodness, that was lonely. I had no idea what to expect in the moments after having her. Staring at her perfect face and fingers was my only solace as my uterus contracted back to a smaller size. Becoming her mother empowered me.

After we had our second daughter, Aurora, I felt the loneliest I'd ever felt. I was a mess after having her. I was scared of juggling two children during the hours my husband would be at work. See, I had Aurora on a Wednesday, and by Monday I was in the car-pool line with Kalima. My husband was back at work. We lived far away from my friends and had rare visitors. I cried a lot.

The one thing I underestimated was the role that resuming a sexual relationship with my husband would have. While I struggled in adjusting to postpartum life with two, it was the strength of my marriage that helped me. But it wasn't easy to get there. Being in pain makes it hard to be happy, feel sexy, or anything positive in truth. Leaking milk and wondering if at the bare minimum my vagina had snapped back really had me insecure.

See, no one talks about sex after baby. I didn't know what to be prepared for. I was awkward, squishy, and filled with milk. But my husband and I talked through what would make me feel comfortable and we took things slow. I began to feel more like myself. And me feeling more like myself enabled me to handle feeling lonely. I began to feel empowered again.

It's not important to everyone, but sex is really important to me. That physical connection bridged a gap with us, and when our third child was born, things were way easier because we had a blueprint.

—Aaronica Cole,
thecrunchymommy.com
(@aaronicabcole)

When I found out I was pregnant with triplets, I knew my body would change, but I was not prepared for how much. My body did miraculous things carrying three babies at one time. It stretched and stretched and allowed me to carry them to our goal date. It still blows my mind that my 105-pound body birthed three nearly five-pound babies at one time. After the babies came, I was in a bit of a postpartum fog, mentally and physically. It took time before I started taking steps for necessary change. And my new body would certainly be one that would take time for me to love all over again. My body was covered in stretch marks and so much loose skin, not to mention even a year and a half after I delivered I had people asking me if I was pregnant again. It took a daily conscious effort to find beauty in my new body. Two years went by before I could fully embrace and celebrate my postpartum body. I finally felt comfortable in my own skin. I found so much beauty in my stretch marks. They were a road map of my journey to Motherhood. The thing is, the woman I was before kids may not have had stretch marks or loose skin, but she did not know how to love herself. And that is the beauty of my own postpartum journey. I have never felt so confident and beautiful in my own skin. I have an appreciation for my body and what it has done to carry life. I chose positive self-talk and learned the beauty in embracing my body for exactly as it is, and that is something no one can take from me.

—Desiree Fortin,
theperfectmom.com
(@theperfectmom)

If a mother wants to share her wrinkly belly, she can. If a mother wants to share her stretch-marked belly, she can. If a mother wants to share her belly full of rolls, she can. If a mother wants to share her excess skin on her belly, she can. If a mother wants to share her C-section scar, she can. Because she is empowered. And no one else's opinion of her will ever be as important and meaningful as her own opinion of her. Just because women don't look alike doesn't mean we aren't all beautiful. This is your reminder to celebrate where you are, as you are, today, tomorrow, and every day moving forward.

MY EXPERIENCE WITH FERTILITY AND FITNESS DURING PREGNANCY AND POSTPARTUM

I've had an irregular menstrual cycle most of my life, but it hadn't resulted in any health concerns until my late twenties, when my weight was at its highest. During that time, I spoke to my doctor about starting a family, a conversation that first sparked me to begin my fitness journey in 2015. I brought up my irregular cycle and shared that I was afraid it might be an issue since my husband, Bobby, and I had never "tried" (but we had also never "not tried") to conceive; I hadn't gotten pregnant in our four years of marriage. At that moment the discussion shifted, as my doctor recommended that I begin losing weight in an effort to possibly help regulate my cycle. I was told that I would also need to be tested for other signs of PCOS (polycystic ovary syndrome), one of the most common female hormone disorders and one of the most common causes of female infertility.

According to the US Department of Health & Human Services Office on Women's Health,[12] PCOS signs include:

- Irregular menstrual cycle
- Excess facial and body hair
- Acne
- Thinning hair or hair loss, male-pattern baldness
- Weight gain

The more time I spent reading about PCOS, irregular cycles, and the difficulties of conceiving, the more terrified I became of not being able to become a birth mother. I was anxious and panicky and refused to talk about it with anyone, not even Bobby. Before this, I had never before pictured a life without kids, and the thought now of that happening was unbearable. I internalized all that fear, blaming myself. It was a constant internal battle of feeling disappointed in my body, mixed with confusion when there were no other signs of PCOS. After blood tests, sonograms, and physical exams, the signs just weren't there outside of weight. I became convinced that my menstrual cycle would most likely regulate once I lost a lot of weight. So, I committed to doing whatever was necessary to make that happen. One year into my fitness journey, I noticed my cycle was more regular. By January 2017, I had six monthly cycles in a row—it felt promising. Although I was still considered plus-size after losing almost a hundred pounds, that February I got pregnant with Maci.

Seeing that positive test result felt both beautiful and overwhelming. I remember constantly thinking, *Wow, it worked!* The weight loss actually worked! Instead of focusing on the habits and behaviors I was adopting (such as regular physical activity), I could only seem to feel thankful for the number that changed on the scale.

I had an entirely healthy pregnancy and gained around sixty pounds during it. Although I continued working out until I was thirty-six weeks pregnant (delivering at thirty-eight weeks after a thirty-hour labor), I still gained weight. That weight gain was at the top of my list of concerns throughout my pregnancy and postpartum experience. It took up a ton of my focus, so much so that I wasn't paying attention to what else was happening with my body and neglected to acknowledge or research the ways in which I could help it heal, not just ways to shrink it back to "normal," as if there were some sort of "reset to factory settings" button.

For most of my pregnancy, I was just obsessed with the number on the scale and neglected to realize that so many other physical and mental factors are at play. There are so many important pieces of information that I wished someone had shared with me during that period, so I'm sharing them here with you.

While there are increased risks during pregnancy for plus-size women, such as gestational diabetes, studies have proven that adopting an active lifestyle can help reduce the risks.[13] But that doesn't mean there aren't ways to focus on adopting these healthy pregnancy behaviors without placing all of our mental energy on the number on the scale.

Some of my favorite activities that are usually safe during pregnancy include:

- **Walking:** A great place to start for anyone new to exercise.
- **Swimming / water aerobics:** The water supports the weight of the baby while taking it easy on joints and muscles. This is especially helpful for those with lower-back pain.
- **Stationary bike:** These are safer than riding a regular bicycle during pregnancy, even with a growing belly. Recumbent bikes are also a great option if a regular stationary bike still feels difficult to get on or off of.
- **Yoga:** Inform your yoga instructor that you're pregnant before class in order for them to help you modify or avoid certain poses. Search in your area for prenatal yoga classes specifically for pregnant women to see what might be available.

- **Strength training:** It's definitely possible to safely continue strength training using weights during pregnancy, but as with all exercise during pregnancy, always consult your health-care provider first.

Signing up for classes or following a specific program is not required to engage in physical activity. Something like dancing in your underwear is just as beneficial and counts just as much. But it's probably best to avoid activities in which you might fall or get hit in the belly, or anything that requires you to lie flat on your back or raise your body temperature a little too high. The best thing you can do is remain hydrated and try paying attention to your body and listening to its cues. Stop any activity that is causing chest pain, dizziness, or anything raising concerns, and be sure to inform your health-care provider as soon as possible if it does.

Although I continued workouts throughout most of my pregnancy, at thirty-six weeks, my doctor and I noticed my blood pressure was slightly higher than normal. So after that, I allowed my body more rest and focused more on light walking rather than body squats and biceps curls. It was empowering to, for one of the very first times, actually listen to my body and honor its needs. Two weeks later, Maci was born after a thirty-hour labor that I'm proud to have had the strength to power through. It's possible to exercise safely during pregnancy; it just takes a little extra listening to our bodies without all of the unnecessary judgment and shame.

Within days of giving birth, I was already planning for the day I would jump right back into exercising. But I felt broken in more ways than one. I was worried about never being able to get back to where I was, and it's a lot of the reason why I internally began to spiral down. I wasn't prepared for just how different I would feel for a while. It was easy to get sucked into the desire to erase any signs of pregnancy. Getting that green light a few weeks postpartum to begin reintroducing exercise felt exciting, for sure. But it wasn't all sunshine and rainbows. All of a sudden, I was squirting everywhere from every angle and everything just felt, well . . . loose, which I now know is completely normal! Remember, even though birth is absolutely beautiful, it's also physically traumatic for a woman's body, which needs time to recover. With other types of injuries, the typical recommendation you might receive from a doctor is six weeks off any normal physical activity, with a slow introduction of rehabilitative exercises to help heal. That's similar to the healing during postpartum. Most women can begin reintroducing movement into their routine anywhere between six to twelve weeks postpartum, but always receive clearance first from your doctor.

Here are a few common postpartum changes that might take some adjusting to when physical activity is reintroduced, and my personal experience navigating them:

- **Sore vagina:** Well, it's more like the area between the vagina and rectum called the perineum, but it feels sore because it stretches and sometimes tears during vaginal births.

  Helpful tips: Try Kegel exercises (squeeze the muscles that you use to stop yourself from peeing and hold those muscles tight for ten seconds and then release), cold packs, and warm baths. Avoid any exercises that require you to sit on a hard surface. Sitting on pillows can be helpful. Be gentle with yourself if you decide to do any running. Try a brisk walk for a while first.

- **Tender boobs:** Whether you're breastfeeding or not, you might be adjusting to a new tenderness and your boobs may be rather leaky.

  Helpful tips: Wear supportive, well-fitted bras. Massage your boobs often and use a warm cloth over any sore areas. Take extra nursing pads and nipple cream everywhere, and don't feel bad when you have to adjust the nursing pads in the middle of any physical activity. Try to breastfeed or pump before you exercise to reduce the discomfort.

- **Stress urinary incontinence:** This basically just means that you may now accidentally pee a little when you laugh or sneeze (as well as anytime you do exercises such as jumping jacks or dead lifts).

  Helpful tips: Wear leakproof underwear during any physical activity. (Yes, those exist and they are amazing!) You can also do pelvic floor exercises to help strengthen your pelvic muscles and possibly experience this less. Pelvic physical therapy is available, whether it's postpartum related or not. You can search for pelvic health professionals in your area at pelvicguru.com.

- **Diastasis recti:** When your ab muscles separate, creating discomfort and pain with certain movements.

  Helpful tips: Try consulting pelvic floor therapists, who can teach you the proper posture and techniques for daily activities and lifting. Following guidelines provided by a pelvic floor therapist can potentially prevent your ab muscles from separating farther, while also incorporating the proper exercises to correct any separation.

- **Stretch marks:** Those tigerlike stripes that appear on such places as our hips, stomach, arms, and boobs when our bodies expand and grow. (These commonly occur in pregnancy, but all people have them because people grow.)

  Helpful tips: If your stretch marks are itchy or physically painful, you can use creams and lotions to help ease any discomfort. The marks may not ever disappear, but they will fade over time. They are normal, and how cool is it that your body stretched and made sure it had room for all of your growth.

- **Hemorrhoids and constipation:** When you struggle pooping and the veins around your butthole get swollen.

  Helpful tips: Try a warm bath, eating lots of fiber, drinking plenty of water, and using over-the-counter ointments and sprays that have been recommended to you by your doctor. Personally, I was never able to exercise through either of these issues because it was too uncomfortable.

A few other things that can happen: temporary hair loss (usually back to normal within a year and nothing that a headband can't handle during workouts for the wild wisps) and lots of sweat and exhaustion. Also, the possibility of perinatal mood disorders, but that deserves its own section, which can be found on page 56.

If you're ever worried about any of these discomforts, especially while exercising, call your health-care provider as soon as possible.

Keep in mind, none of these postpartum changes are the "price of motherhood" that you have to pay when you become a mom. These changes should not feel like consequences because they aren't. It doesn't help that postnatal care can sometimes feel dismissive of these issues, labeling them "motherhood side effects" and sending you on your way after a six-week postpartum checkup. So, it's normal that you just assume the previous forms of exercise that you used to love just won't work for you anymore. I know that a part of you might feel like you've lost your identity during this massive change. But I hope you know that you are capable, even when you feel like you're not, and even when everything feels like it is too much. And I hope that you know you are significant. Even when it feels like you're not.

If you're like me, you'll feel frustrated with getting back into the old fitness routine while experiencing lots of these changes. That's normal, but remember that your body created life and deserves some time to heal. Not only that, it deserves food, nourishment, and a whole lot of grace. One of the best ways to ease back into a little bit of exercise is to perform core-focused stretching and mobility exercises. I know that these aren't exciting and might not feel like "working out," but they will be extremely helpful for healing and recovery. So many wonderful women have designed incredible pregnancy- and postpartum-focused workout guides, some even specializing in areas such as diastasis recti. Some of my favorites can be found in the "Additional Resources" section of this book. Once you feel a bit more comfortable, you can begin exploring the "A" option exercises in my Twelve-Week Strength Training Guide, found in Part 5 on page 111.

And for more plus-size pregnancy/postpartum fitness, fertility, and motherhood resources, please see page 197.

MATERNAL MENTAL HEALTH

One in five adults suffers from a mental illness. I am one of them. I have struggled with my anxiety and depression for years and first began noticing intrusive thoughts when I was in middle school. I never told anyone at the time, but I felt scared often. It never occurred to me that I could have a mental illness. During my senior year of high school, I felt a major shift in my mental health that I didn't quite know how to explain to family and friends. I felt fearful a lot of the time, and my body image was deteriorating. I never mentioned to anyone the intrusive thoughts I was experiencing and was confused as to why I felt such a deep, dark pain. Not until I began self-harming and attempted suicide did my family become alarmed. My memory of this time as I finished the remainder of my senior year is mostly fuzzy, but it was the most isolating time of my life. I started my first semester of college and eventually stopped refilling my prescription and attending therapy while continuing to live a life filled with shame. After my suicide attempt, I'd spent time in an adolescent unit, went to therapy, and first started taking medication. When I got to college, I never spoke of that period in my life because it felt as if I could finally move forward and tuck the past into where I felt it belonged. I pretended for a long time that my mental illness wasn't real. I figured I was just out there, a little crazy, and simply couldn't handle my emotions. When I was pregnant, I remember thinking that there was just no way I would get postpartum depression. Even though I had dealt with depression my entire life, it didn't make sense to me that having a baby would make me depressed. I wondered why women I knew felt so depressed after having their baby, especially women who had never seemed depressed before. I assumed that achieving my dream of becoming a mom would be the last thing to trigger my anxiety and depression.

Throughout my pregnancy, I imagined sharing an incredible bond with my baby, one that included breastfeeding. Not long after Maci was born, those dreams quickly turned cold as she struggled to latch. I felt myself being pulled into the depression quicksand and fought it with everything I had. But the harder I fought, the more I sank. I felt anger toward my body for gaining weight and for not allowing Maci to latch. I felt anxious with every failed attempt. I felt weak because I was exhausted and just needed a break. I felt ashamed because I assumed I wasn't strong enough to handle any of this. So I went silent and pretended that I was okay. Every time I held Maci in my arms, I would stare down at her, so in love and yet simultaneously so ashamed. Because in those weeks, I felt that she could do better than me.

I knew I needed help, but I spent months avoiding my truth, assuming it would mean I was somehow admitting that I couldn't handle being a mom, much less a good one. I would calmly say I was a little too tired for that outing we got invited to again. When what I wanted to say was that I was terrified to step foot out of the house because I was scared that I would fail my daughter. I wanted to say that I was worried, overwhelmed, and straight-up terrified, but I still kept silent because I felt like a failure to admit that motherhood wasn't bringing me joy and fulfillment. I felt the most alone I have ever felt in my life. What it took for me to speak up was one terrifying moment in the shower, when I felt my eyes scanning around for what would help me take away my pain. Panic took over and I grasped the towel rack, doing everything possible to stop these spiraling feelings of shame, sadness, and unworthiness. It took everything in me to just breathe. Then in what felt like the first time in my life, I chose me. Still wet, I walked into our bedroom and sat next to Bobby. I told him, for the first time, that I wasn't okay. And he listened. Not long after, I found myself sobbing in the living room of my parents' house in front of my family as they promised to help. For the first time, I felt seen for who I was: a woman who deserves love, help, and support.

I didn't get on medication right away. As of this writing, I'm still trying to get back on medication for my anxiety and depression since doctors want to treat my "obesity" before prescribing any medication. The weight stigma associated with my medical care has been a difficult experience for me, especially for my mental health. But medication wasn't exactly new for me. I knew medication and therapy were both self-care items that would help, but I had never seen them normalized and openly discussed for someone of my weight. Until I found myself as a new mother, off medication, assuming these would be the happiest moments of my life when it would be the last thing I would need. I'm hopeful that my options for medication will be available soon, and it won't make me any less of a good mom if I get on meds. Ironically enough, the moment I did finally feel like a good mom was the moment I decided to ask for help and open up about my experiences to Bobby. This eventually led me to completely open up on social media and my blog about my most vulnerable mental health moments.

I began connecting with so many other women and mothers who also experienced many different types of mood disorders. It was quickly becoming a main topic of discussion across my social media platforms. By August of 2019, Bobby and I received an invite to visit the AHN Alexis Joy D'Achille Center for Perinatal Mental Health in Pittsburgh for the first-ever #MyWishForMoms Summit, a two-day event that brought together a small group of women in a safe space to discuss our real-life experiences, struggles, and solutions. For the first time Bobby publicly spoke out about his experiences witnessing and preparing for my panic attacks and suicidal thoughts. We had spent most of the first day listening to the stories of women who experienced a perinatal mood and anxiety disorder (PMAD). Bobby would squeeze my hand a little tighter each time another woman bravely shared her story that felt all too familiar for him. I knew it would be a hard conversation for him to have, and when he completely broke down in front of an auditorium full of women who had all experienced something similar to my experience, it became clear that these types of issues are not discussed enough by men. It was one of our most emotional experiences as a couple, but also one of the most alarming to learn the facts and statistics. While exact rates are unknown, here are some generally agreed-upon figures about the number of women who experience postpartum depression:

- One in five women will experience a maternal mental health illness, such as postpartum depression or anxiety.[14]
- In the United States each year, more than eight hundred thousand women will suffer from a pregnancy or postpartum mental health illness.[15]
- Only 15 percent of women with PMADs are diagnosed and will receive treatment.[16]
- A major reason that families don't seek help is because of the stigma associated with postpartum depression and other mental health illnesses.[17]

- More than 20 percent of postpartum deaths are caused by suicide, the most common cause of mortality in postpartum women.[18]
- Women who have a PMAD are 50 percent more likely to have it with their next pregnancy than women who have never had a PMAD.[19]
- African American women suffer from PMAD at rates 35 percent higher than the rest of the population.[20]
- Women in their childbearing years are the largest group with depression in the United States.

These stats make it clear that many women suffer in the aftermath of giving birth. This is why it's even more infuriating that there's so much societal pressure on postpartum women to immediately start exercising and snap right back to normal both physically *and* mentally. While physical fitness is definitely helpful for overall health as postpartum healing and recovery begins, taking care of your mental health can be just as, if not more, important. It could be lifesaving.

To a mother fighting to get her pre-baby body back, while facing inner struggles, I would say, You have not failed as a mother or as a partner. You have not failed as a sister or a teacher or a woman on this earth. You have not failed if you asked for help or because you are now on medication. You have not failed because you just needed a few days away by yourself. You have not failed because you suffered from postpartum depression or anxiety or any mental illness. You have not failed because you got frustrated and raised your voice or because you hid in the closet crying. You have not failed because you missed another workout and can't even think about that yet. The days and hours and minutes might feel hard. They might feel lonely. Your head might get clouded with endless thoughts filled with shame and sadness. But you have not failed. You are not defined by a diagnosis, by your past, or by your most vulnerable moments. You have not failed because you are still here. Because you are stronger than you give yourself credit for. You are braver than you'd like to admit. You will get through this. Because you were never a failure.

Admitting that it's hard or that you're scared or that you're overwhelmed doesn't make you any less than. It doesn't make you unfit to be a mother. It doesn't make you unworthy. All it does is make you human.

For more maternal mental health resources, please see page 194.

WHAT OUR CHILDREN SEE

My daughter is the reason I first even considered exploring fitness through a self-love and body-confident approach. I couldn't even begin to imagine her ever crying on a scale and skipping any of her life's special moments because of that number. Or because any of her physical features weren't within the realm of what's societally accepted. I didn't want her to go through what I went through, what countless other women have gone through.

The 2017 Dove Global Girls Beauty and Confidence Report[21] examined the impact of body esteem, pressures, and confidence on girls everywhere and found:

- Over half of girls around the world do not have high body-esteem.
- Many Generation Zers feel anxious about their appearance, with 45 percent saying they feel more anxious about that than their career prospects or money.
- Eight in ten girls with low body confidence opt out of important life activities, such as engaging with friends and loved ones, due to worrying about the way they look.
- Seven in ten girls stop themselves from eating when they don't feel good about the way they look.
- Low body-esteem and anxieties over appearance are stopping young people from being their best selves, affecting their health, friendships, and even performance at school.

If I was going to reframe Maci's perspective of self-worth from this, I was going to have to teach her that so many other parts about her have purpose. I would need to battle those statistics head-on. She would need to somehow discover that she has more to offer the world than her appearance. She would need to believe that her hopes and dreams and talents make her beautifully special and unique. To do this, I would need to teach her to hold herself in high esteem, to not see fitness as punishment, and to embrace her body. I would need to teach her all the things that I didn't know when I was growing up.

As of this writing, it's been almost three years since I had my daughter and first started constantly searching for any answer to how she might have a chance at loving herself. I knew what had to happen first though: I would have to learn how to love myself. That terrified me to my core because what if I just couldn't do it? Would this mean that it would be impossible for her, too? This thought was one of the things that kept me up at night in the beginning of my postpartum depression. But those swirling thoughts on the topic, which you might have, too, are a result of diet culture, of years of being obsessed with how we look. So even when it's difficult to explore these new ideas, that they are even being given the chance to be explored is huge. Be proud of that.

Here are some ideas for moms wanting to demonstrate high self-esteem to their kids, especially their daughters:

- Go swimming. Wear the swimsuit and get in the pool with your kids without making any unnecessary comments about the way your body looks in your swimsuit. (Unless you're mentioning how much of a hot mama you are, because *duh*.)
- Compliment her often on things that aren't related to the way she looks, such as how creative or talented she is. She's obviously adorable and cute and all of those things that you physically see, but the idea is to help her understand that she is so much more than that.
- When she is old enough, have an honest conversation about beauty distortion in the media. Show her examples of manipulated images next to their original images to help her realize that what she sees on TV, in movies, or in magazines is rarely representative of reality. Remind her that because of this manipulation, it's just not worth making comparisons.

- When she asks you if she's fat or calls someone else fat, try not to give the word *fat* any sort of value. Talk about how all bodies have fat and that the amount that any human has varies from person to person for a variety of reasons. Inform her that the amount of fat on someone's body isn't an indicator of the person's health or worth.
- Avoid saying "I'm so out of shape" or "I feel fat" when you mean that you're feeling tired or stressed-out. Saying either of those phrases implies that you need to be in a certain shape for you to no longer feel those things, which isn't true. If you hear your child saying either of those phrases, ask her if she can explain what she is really feeling and not what she looks like.
- Let her see you enjoying life during moments that you don't have on makeup or a styled outfit. Also, try not to mention or make note of the differences in how you look when you have all of that on again. Commenting that you, or any other woman, look better in makeup or fancy clothes will make her think that she needs those things to be beautiful. Allow her to see style/fashion/makeup as a creative outlet, if she chooses, and not as a requirement of being a woman.
- Show her what different types of bodies look like, including athletes of all sizes, ages, and skin types. Talk frequently about the nonphysical strengths that they need, including mental toughness, self-discipline, determination, and leadership skills.

I know how it can feel like she's going to see all of your imperfections and just not understand. I know that you worry that she will see the size of your body and compare it to the media images of the perfect mom, where you feel as though you'll always fall short. But, you know what? When sharing my shifting perspectives about weight and self-worth, I am constantly met with criticism from strangers on the internet. "But what about the children? What will they see?" they ask. A daughter will see her mother. She will see happiness and love. She will see pride and worth. She will see power and strength. She will see her mama's belly that bounces up and down while doing push-ups like a badass. And seeing these things will show her that physical appearance has nothing to do with worth. That she is so much more than what she looks like or how much she weighs. She will see her body for more than something to just be looked at and manipulated. And maybe, just maybe, I'll give her the chance to think, *Wow, I have such a powerful mother. I must be powerful, too.*

For more body image resources, please see page 194.

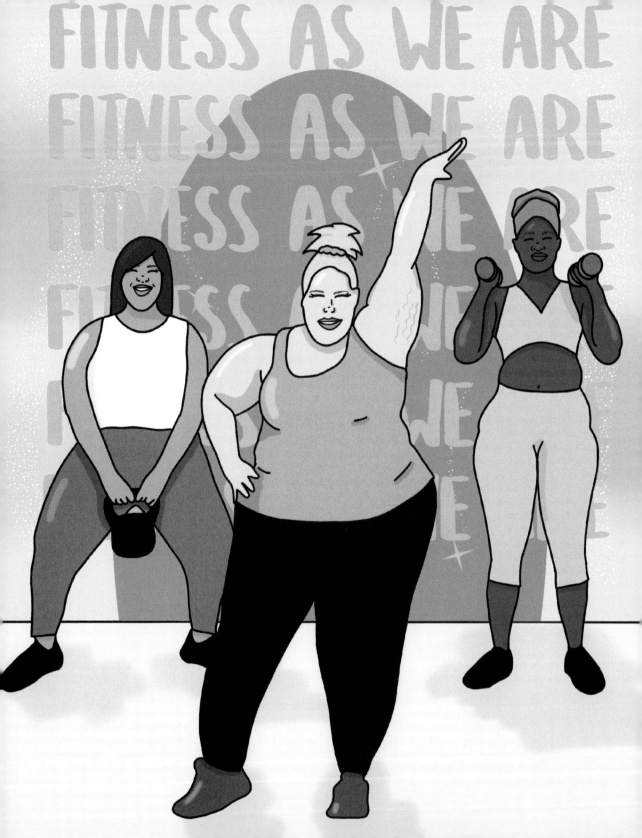

Part 4

The Part Where We Embrace Fitness as We Are

THE BIG WHY

A question for you: If working out, exercising, or any other term you prefer to use for moving your body didn't do anything to alter your appearance . . . would you still do it? Think about that for a moment. Because exercising should be about more than your physical appearance. Sure, exercising might physically change your body in some ways. But it also might not, and that's okay. The benefits of movement extend far beyond an aesthetic. I've been doing all sorts of booty exercises during my training, and you know what? My booty is still the shape of an *H* and is definitely not "Instagram round," but it's a real strong booty that allows me to do all of my favorite heavy lifts. And that's what gives me happiness. That's what gives me my motivation. The "in shape," fit ideal that is constantly advertised or praised isn't necessarily a physical shape. So you shouldn't look toward it as an end goal or the source of your drive. The motivation you're constantly searching for can only be found after you get going, and getting going has to stem from an intention rooted in self-respect, self-worth, confidence, and empowerment. Exercise should be something you enjoy, not an intense, grueling punishment for the food you ate. A lot of us might think that having a different body will cure our bad body image, but a bad body image will only begin to heal once it begins to feel comforted.

Ask yourself these questions before beginning or continuing to explore your relationship with exercise and fitness:

- Do I enjoy this type of movement?
- Am I using exercise as punishment for what I ate or specifically to "earn" my food?
- Does working out feel like a chore?
- Can I finish the sentence "I want to get healthier because ___" with something that isn't my appearance?
- Am I distracted by how I look while I'm working out rather than focusing on my workout?
- Am I missing out on and/or denying life experiences to avoid missing a workout?
- Are there any other tools I can use to manage my stress/anxiety should exercise not be available?
- Why am I choosing to exercise and what am I hoping to gain that doesn't have anything to do with my looks?
- Are the goals that I've set for myself realistic for me financially, logistically, and mentally right now?

SHIFT YOUR FITNESS FOCUS FROM APPEARANCE BASED TO BODY POSITIVE

Choose forms of movement that are fun and enjoyable for you.

If you don't like running, then don't go for a run! There are so many different ways to move our bodies. From group sports to pole dancing to dog walks to swimming to strength training, the list is essentially endless. If you're not sure what you'll like, give a few different things a try and see what makes you smile. If something isn't enjoyable for you, it's not something you should feel bad about! There's nothing wrong with you for not liking an activity that many others do, and it shouldn't discourage you from exploring other options. Finding something you absolutely love doing is going to make your fitness experience fun! Because exercising should be fun. Because fitness is more than a bunch of before and after photos. Because even if we all worked out exactly the same, ate exactly the same, slept exactly the same, and did every single thing the exact same way, all of our bodies would still look different. So, remind yourself that you're more than your body and choose a form of movement that brings you joy and health of the mind, body, and soul. You can't photograph the transformation of what happens inside.

Work out in clothes that are comfortable.

If you're constantly adjusting your clothes and worried about how you'll look in them, your experience will be less enjoyable. Not only that, but you'll constantly be fixated on how you look, rather than how you feel. For example, I stuck with wearing superbaggy clothes when I first started working out because I didn't want my stomach and arm rolls to show or the cellulite on my thighs to be visible through my leggings. It was so fucking hard to move around with those heavy, baggy clothes that always got in my damn way.

When I decided to cut off all the sleeves and midsections of my tees and squat in crop tops and leggings, it was to finally give my body well-deserved comfort instead of making an empowered fashion statement.

Think about how you feel while you're working out, not about how you hope working out will make you look.

I know it's damn near impossible to contemplate anything other than the big secret hidden deep down about why you're even moving your body in the first place (especially when it's something you don't even enjoy doing). But instead of calculating the number of calories you have left to burn in the next ten minutes, try thinking about how your heart is pumping. It's kind of incredible how your body knows exactly what to do when you're exercising, and that it is doing everything possible to help you achieve your goals. Your heart is pumping, your lungs are expanding, your muscles are stretching, and your sweat is dripping to cool you down. At the same time, your stamina, strength, and endurance are all increasing. It's incredible. Make sure to say thank-you when it's over. Your body is badass.

Don't overdo it.

Whether it's because you rely on working out to relieve stress, or because you're feeling that you can never miss a workout for fear of gaining weight, don't overexercise. Our bodies need rest and time to recover from any type of movement. If you tend to push yourself too hard when exercising, consider checking in with yourself frequently through either journal prompts from the list of questions above or a simple peaceful moment of reflection. Listen to your body and stop if you're in pain or fatigued. There's nothing to be ashamed of for needing a moment of rest or ending the session for the day. Fitness isn't "all or nothing," and you know your body better than anyone else.

Explore fitness intuitively without a focus on weight loss, especially if you're trying to focus on your health.

Weight loss isn't a magic gateway to achieving peak health. Weight loss can stem from numerous other factors—including genetics, weight stigma, eating disorders, chronic illnesses—that aren't healthy. Even if you're aiming to achieve certain aesthetics, think realistically about where your motivation or "body goals" are coming from. Consider any previous body-obsession patterns you've experienced and how they may have impacted you. There's nothing wrong with wanting a six-pack, but it might be something to tread carefully around if you have experience with any type of body-dysmorphic thoughts. Be sure to create boundaries for yourself and move your body in ways that feel good. Some days you'll be able to push a little harder, and some days you'll need to be gentler. Also, consider taking off the fitness tracker for a workout and trust how you feel more than what the data might show if you find it distracting you and negatively impacting your workout. Focusing on supplemental health-promoting behaviors such as drinking more water, prioritizing sleep, and utilizing stress-management tools will most likely be far more beneficial to your health than compulsively checking calories burned throughout every workout. And, hey! This might not even apply to you. Maybe you're not tapping away and distracted by your watch during workouts or mentally drained by all the beeping alerts. You know your body and mind best, so you know when something might be hurting you more than it's helping. Be willing to listen and adjust safely when that happens.

Choose goals that have nothing to do with how you look.

Measuring your progress and setting goals can be about so much more than pounds or inches lost. There are a lot of different ways to set goals and measure progress, from strength (dead-lift PR, anyone?); to endurance (5K fun run, anyone?); to flexibility (toe touching for easier shoe tying, anyone?); to speed (spin class sprints, anyone?); to just straight-up creating joy. Taking the focus away from a constant pressure to appear different will create room for growth in other areas just as meaningful. I love setting weekly goals that focus on what I'm hoping to lift on bench, squat, and dead lift. Sometimes it's a simple set of triples at a weight I've already lifted, and sometimes it's a personal record I'm hoping to achieve. It can be soul cleansing to measure your progress through what your body can do rather than how your body is admired.

Choose a trainer and/or fitness studio that is body positive and weight inclusive, rather than weight-centric.

If you choose to engage a personal trainer, you have some options and should talk to multiple people. Here are some examples of a few body-positive questions to ask when interviewing a potential trainer:

- Will you be prioritizing my well-being over my weight loss?
- Will there be a requirement to measure my body or take photos?
- If I'm not comfortable working out in front of a mirror yet, will I have the option to avoid it until I'm ready?
- Will we be able to set goals that are more focused on how I'm feeling rather than how my body looks?

Read reviews and testimonials from some of the trainer's previous clients. Trainers' websites should clearly state their body-positive values. Their social media content should celebrate movement beyond how it can alter appearance. But above all else, in choosing trainers, whether they claim to be body positive or not, ask yourself if you feel welcome in their facility. Once you've started working with them, monitor if they listen to your goals and design a program that feels right for your body. Make sure they respectfully answer questions about any of the exercises that they have assigned to you and create modifications as needed, without making negative comments about your body or capabilities. If you're searching for body-positive trainers (both in person and online), I suggest using the Super Fit Hero Body Positive Fitness Finder online.

Unfollow all social media accounts that are triggering for you and do a full social media cleanse.

Even if it's friends or family that you're uncomfortable unfollowing, hit the mute button for a while if their posts are currently triggering. Fill your feed with people of all shapes and sizes, living and thriving and empowered as they are. Think of it this way: if it's constantly making you feel like shit about yourself, it sure as hell doesn't deserve to live rent-free on your feed.

For body-positive trainers and fitness accounts to follow, see page 201.

SAYING YES TO THE GYM
(AND EVERYTHING ELSE YOU LOVE)

I'll never forget the feeling of picking up my first set of heavy weights. Through the mirror, I saw my body—the one I had hated for so long and forced onto treadmills for punishment—show me just what it could do. Back then, only the bar sat at the top of my back. And damn did it feel good. I think that's the moment when I knew I had found a way to move my body that brought me enjoyment and a sense of empowerment, without thoughts of how my outer appearance would/could/might change. This was something I had never experienced before. For the first time, I took a moment to say thank you to my body for what it could do, rather than criticizing it for all that it could not. The rocky road toward this internal dialogue hasn't always been easy, but it's been worth every tough, intentional moment of redirecting my mind-set toward it.

Just before our family moved from Houston to Fort Worth, my mom and I were both attending Camp Gladiator outdoor group-fitness workouts near her house in Fort Worth. Camp Gladiator is a company that runs boot-camp/all-level–style classes that focus on strength, endurance, and high-intensity interval training. My mom was so excited to introduce me to her trainer, Shane Phillips, who was also training her to powerlift! That was always my favorite part about Camp Gladiator: you could travel to an entirely different city and still get the chance to work out with an amazing trainer. So, during Thanksgiving break in 2016, Shane invited me to join a group for a powerlifting training session at his personal studio while I was in Fort Worth. It was my first experience with powerlifting. I tried not to make a big deal about it at the time, but I was hooked. I had never experienced that kind of happiness before while exercising. It was exciting as hell.

When I got back to Houston, I brought it up with my CG trainer after the holidays, which is when she agreed to send me some simple lifting workouts to try in a gym. By February 2017 I'd signed up for a gym membership, but it wasn't a great experience. I was neck-deep in my disordered eating and obsession with exercising. So many intimidating "bros" were around the gym that I got cut off just about every time I tried grabbing an available squat rack. But when I did get my hands on a barbell, it was exhilarating. The feeling was indescribable and like nothing any other movement had ever made me feel. Within a month, I discovered that I was pregnant. Bobby and I had to make a financial decision. I quit my job and we packed up our things to move in with my parents in Fort Worth around April 2017, and I continued Camp Gladiator with Shane throughout all of my pregnancy. I knew I would be giving it a try again at his studio once I was cleared to work out postpartum. And that's exactly what I did. For a year and a half, from January 2018 until June 2019, I attended both Camp Gladiator workouts and powerlifting sessions at Shane's studio. Throughout this time, my views and feelings around exercise and fitness were shifting. I was beginning to crave the positive feeling that exercise gave me over the fluctuations in my weight. The summer of 2019, Shane invited me and a few other women who trained with him to attend a yoga class. After the yoga class, we all went out for margaritas on the patio. It was one of the first times I opened up to him about how powerlifting and embracing fitness with this new mind-set made me feel. I could tell he didn't completely understand, but he never questioned me. A few weeks later, he asked to meet me at the gym to get a workout in together. The actual gym, not his studio. He stood by me as I signed the paperwork and interrupted the guy behind the desk, who was preparing to ask me a million questions about my weight-loss goals. It was the first time I said out loud, "I'm a powerlifter," and I let him know that I don't need any of their extra services. It was incredibly empowering. But I was officially back at the gym. And this time was different.

From that day until around March 2020, when all gyms suddenly closed due to COVID-19 (they are still closed as I write this), I walked into the gym to train with Shane as a lifting partner. Every exercise we did, I asked questions and he always had answers. I noticed patterns in the way he formatted our workouts and constantly paid attention to his directions. I always felt that I was probably annoying with how much I would ask. But my curiosity stemmed from how much I loved the feeling working out like this gave me. I always wanted to know more. And it geniunely felt fun. That's how I knew it was the right kind of exercise for me. During that time, I hit PRs that I never thought possible, competed in my first powerlifting meet, competed in my first combine event, and was invited to Under Armour headquarters as an athlete for their 2020 Human Performance Summit. All because I finally stopped allowing my fear of the gym and working out in public to continue holding me back.

I know reading this makes the process sound easy, but I also know just how uncomfortable that first day ever (or first day back) might feel. So let's walk through it, shall we? And maybe the next time, you'll remember this example of how to create a mind-set shift.

You walk into the gym. (Or any new place where you'll be moving your body in front of others.) You always wonder if everyone is looking. You glance in the mirror and make awkward eye contact with a stranger and quickly look away.

Well, crap, you think loudly.

Now they see me. I wonder what they thought.

I'm not good enough.

My body is not strong enough.

My body is not capable.

My body is disgusting.

No one wants to see this.

Why do I always do this? Okay. Calm down. Breathe. And now you can't stop thinking about why you even came.

Then you look down at your yoga mat. Or the dumbbells. Or whatever and wherever you decided to show up for today. You take another deep breath. And you remember.

This isn't about them. It's not about what anyone can see. It's not about your squishy belly. Or your dimples showing through your leggings or the rolls on your arms. It's never been about any of those things. It's just about you. Your mind might be hard to convince in the beginning. That body of yours might be hard to bend at first. But that soul of yours? Well, it's been waiting your whole life for this. And that's when you smile. You breathe in and accept this moment. It's okay to be seen. The world is glad that you exist. Put your energy into that truth, not into the lies you have continued to internalize on repeat. It's not your fault that you've been programmed to believe so many lies. It's okay for you to be seen. It's okay for you to do hard things. It's okay for you to exist in your current body. (I mean, we can't get too comfortable in it anyway. It's going to keep changing and adjusting itself for us for the rest of our lives, which is beautiful when you think about it.) It's okay for you to look different because different has never meant wrong. And it's okay for you to struggle accepting all of this for what it's been all along—the truth.

I wish that I could go back and tell my younger self so many things. But instead I'll tell you: It's not your fault that you're treated differently because of your body size. The way you're mocked, left out of most clothing-brand sizing, rarely ever represented anywhere, and forced to strive for thinness at all costs has nothing to do with your worth. You are more than a body, and that body is going to disrupt a lot of that toxic societal energy by simply showing up. So, do all of the shit you love and keep on showing up—especially when it feels scary and uncomfortable. That's always going to offer your greatest opportunity for growth.

STRENGTH TRAINING AND WHY I'M OBSESSED

I didn't begin strength training to break records. I didn't have some grand plan to ever write a book about my experiences with it or to be someone who found herself through it. But here I am. Strength training and powerlifting has taught me a lot about myself, about how I see the world, and about how much strength I've always had. I discovered that I didn't need to break records or have some grand plan to benefit immensely from strength training. All I needed to do was just embrace it.

What exactly is strength training?

Also known as resistance training or weight training, strength training is a type of physical exercise designed to increase strength. Simply put, strength training uses either your body weight or other weighted/resistance tools such as dumbbells, kettlebells, resistance bands, or barbells. And, no, strength training won't immediately make you look like a bulky body-builder, unless you want to.

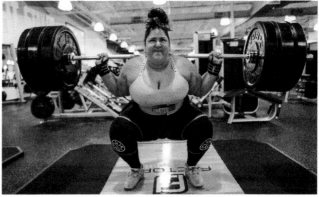

A lot of misconceptions are out there, one of which is that strength training is simple. It is actually a quite difficult and an ex-tremely slow process, especially for women. Further, the fitness world seems to fuel misconceptions sur-rounding the word *strength* and what it refers to. With all that, it makes sense why beginners are so intimidated, because when we hear the phrase *strength training*, we can't help but think of the Hulk. But (eye roll) it's not just the Hulk that benefits from being strong. All humans could benefit from increasing their strength.

Here are just a few reasons why strength training has been so beneficial for me, and why I feel it's important (especially for women) to lift some heavy shit:

- **Increased confidence and self-esteem!** Seriously, I talk about this all the time, but it's because it has been so damn true in my experience. Witnessing what my body can do has given me such a big confidence boost. You want to feel empowered? Pick up any size weight and witness the magic that is within you, one that flows through your muscles and bones and heart and all the way deep down into your soul. Isn't it beautiful? Release all of the assumptions that confidence is only ever found through a lower number on the scale or on the label of your jeans. The magic has always been there, waiting for you to let it out.

- **Stronger muscles, joints, heart, and body!** The beauty of our strength is tucked away in places of our bodies that we just can't see, but will forever be something we can feel. It's there in the way we walk, the way we run in the backyard with our kids, the way we bend over to pick something up off the floor, and throughout our entire human experience. Studies have found that strength training for just thirty minutes twice a week will improve our functional performance, bone density, strength, heart health, and muscle health as we age.[22] It's never too late to show your muscles, joints, heart, and bones a little love by picking up some weights! Even adding in some movements that use your body weight as resistance instead of weights can be just as effective. (For example, squatting onto a chair, stepping up and down on the first step of stairs, lunges, or push-ups.)

- **Lower risk for injuries!** The more strength we build in our muscles, the lower the risk we have for falling, tripping, or stumbling doing everyday tasks. It also allows our bodies to be more resistant to injuries, including any general aches and pains. When I started strength training, I noticed that I was less clumsy, as I avoided tripping over a toy only to hop over it just fine, which wouldn't have happened before. For the first time, I had a lot of control over my body and its everyday movements.

- **Improves sleep quality!** I have always struggled with my sleep. Moving my body and building strength has made me sleep better, as I can lie in bed at night with a clearer mind. The way our brains release those wonderful "feel good" chemicals, known as endorphins, during strength training is a beautiful miracle. They not only give us the feeling of confidence and empowerment but also an opportunity to relieve anxiety and stress. When you don't feel anxious or stressed, you can get a better night's sleep.

- **Better overall quality of life!** I can't emphasize it enough. The confidence, the health benefits, happiness boost, and the overall growth of my mind, body, and soul that I get from strength training have given me life in times that life felt almost unbearably not worth living. Through strength training, I discovered my own worth. And it turned out, I'm a total badass.

Now that we've cleared up why it's amazing and incredibly beneficial for all bodies to incorporate strength-training exercises, let's discuss how you can do it safely. Whether you're new to strength training or just need a refresher before you grab your next size up in weights, here are all of my best training tips to set you up for success on your journey toward all those future strength gains:

- **Safety first, always.** From the dumbbell size you choose to your lifting form to your breathing technique, it's so important to keep the golden rule of safety first at the forefront of your mind.
- **Always warm up and cool down.** Stretch and get your heart pumping before diving straight into a workout. I usually aim for about five minutes of stretching and mobility before and after a workout. I've included a simple warm-up and cooldown in Part 5 alongside my Twelve-Week Strength Training Guide. Whether you use it or not, remember to move and stretch your body in one way or another both before and after your workouts. It's important for your muscles' recovery and will certainly help prevent injuries.
- **When starting, choose a weight that is lighter and increase the weight slowly over time.** This is known as progressive overload and is the key to building strength over time! It can be difficult at first to find the right-size weights, which is why starting small will be the most helpful and safe. It's okay if you're not sure what low might even mean for you. Grab a five-pound or eight-pound weight, try a few reps, and adjust from there from how you feel. (It's totally okay to start without weights if the five-pound weights are still a little too heavy. Only you know what feels the best for you, but just know that at whatever pace you progress, you're a total badass!) You will eventually be able to increase the weight that you're lifting, but it's important to take this slowly. Listen to your

body and only increase in small increments, between two to five pounds at a time. While working your way through my training guide, you can reevaluate your weights at the beginning of weeks 4, 7, and 10 during A Workouts.

For example, if you used 10-pound weights from weeks 1 to 3, consider trying one or two sets using 12-pound weights and the remaining sets using the 10-pound weights during the first workout of week 4. If you're finishing all of the sets and feeling as if you could have done another set, continue using the heavier 12-pound weights until the next weight reevaluation. However, if you started at a lower weight than you probably needed to, you may end up moving up weights sooner. This is a unique experience, so remember to always listen to your body and adjust your weights (in either direction) as needed!

- **Weight-selection pro tip:** When trying to determine the right weight, try 10 reps of the exercise. If you reach 10 and feel that you could easily have done a few more, the weight is too light. If you only get to 3 to 4 reps before reaching failure, the weight is too heavy. (The same holds true if the exercise requires 5 reps. The weight is too light if you could have done up to 10 reps, and it's too heavy if you couldn't quite make it to 2 reps before reaching failure.) Oh, and *failure* isn't a bad word. It's just a general descriptor for reaching the point of muscle exhaustion and not being able to complete a rep. Never be ashamed of reaching failure. It's usually a fantastic learning moment because the day *will* come when you complete it and you'll remember that previous time you didn't quite get it!

- **Document your reps and the size of weights you used for each workout along with how it felt during it.** I love tracking my progress in a workout log. It's extremely helpful when deciding whether to move up in weights. This can simply be within the notes apps on your phone as I do or through other apps such as Strong. There's no right or wrong way to track (should you choose to), and it's definitely not a requirement. It's just one way to track how you're doing on the road to all of those potential gains. (Can I get a "Hell yeah!"?)

- **Always focus on using proper lifting form/technique.** This is what will increase your strength by safely working all of the right muscles! Using bad or incorrect form increases injury risks, so pay attention to which muscles each exercise is intended to work. It will always be more beneficial to lift a lighter weight with proper form than to lift a heavier weight with bad form. If you're finding yourself swaying and using your entire body to lift a weight that's intended to work your biceps, it's probably too heavy! The more you focus on the muscle groups you're training by using proper form, the more you'll begin to notice an increase in your power. Also, take your time with every rep. Rushing through reps and sets isn't going to be very beneficial. Slowing it down is going to help you isolate the muscles you're working and prevent you from relying on any momentum to lift the weight. (This is why I first started recording my training sessions. It was an easy way for me to check my form and ensure that I wasn't relying on momentum. I eventually started sharing the recordings on my Instagram stories, and I guess you could say the rest is history!)

- **Pay attention to your breathing during lifts.** Always remember to breathe! Make sure to breathe in and out normally and comfortably to establish a rhythm. Try breathing out while lifting the weight and breathing in while lowering it. It takes time to practice and find a rhythm that works best for you. Just make sure you keep on breathing!

- **Take rest days when you need them, not just when your training program tells you to.** I say this a lot, but it's because I mean it: listen to your body. It won't hurt you one bit to take a few days off to recover if you're in pain. The old "no pain, no gain" saying is outdated and should not dictate how you approach your fitness experience. It's not all or nothing. Do what you can, when you can. No matter what, you're killing it and I'm proud of you.

THE PUSH-UPS POSSIBILITIES

Think of all the times that someone in your life has told you to just do "girl push-ups." You know, all those awkward moments you may have noticed when an instructor (or that one PE teacher) encouraged you to do push-ups on your knees, enthusiastically shouting, "It's okay if you need to do girl push-ups instead!"—as if that were somehow motivational to hear. (Eyes roll back so far you see your backyard.) Now throw that term in the trash where it belongs. Because *girl push-ups* (or any other variations on the term) are just modified push-ups for anyone who needs a little assistance. Having to start out with these push-ups is no big deal! All people, at one point or another, couldn't do push-ups on their toes, and many athletes still use modifications once getting up on their toes becomes possible. It's all normal! But your gender or sexual identity has nothing to do with your fitness capabilities.

I once believed that I'd never be able to execute full push-ups, but after about a year of upper-body strength training, I was suddenly doing push-ups in a full plank off my toes. To get there, I didn't focus on doing push-ups every single day to improve my form. I just started focusing more on developing strength in my shoulders, chest, back, and core. (Another reason I love strength training: it gave me the chance to try push-ups on my toes!) I was reaching for my push-up goals long before the moment I ever thought I would be able to. Suddenly, I was doing them on one leg and balancing on medicine balls for an extra challenge.

Seeing my body able to do these incredible exercises, I stopped believing two false narratives: that I needed to modify my exercises; and that once I stopped using the modifications sometimes, I would no longer ever need them. Now I know that it's okay to do push-ups up on my toes when I can, and also to do other variations when I can. (My husband sometimes spots me doing push-ups on the kitchen counter now, so it's possible to get your exercises in anywhere!)

Both push-ups with and without modifications are beneficial, and either choice is just as good for you as the other. So, before you count yourself out, give yourself the chance to give up that old, washed-up narrative. Strength training will naturally develop the muscles you need to master the push-up, so I encourage you to incorporate strength exercises into your routine, as that is a sure way to move toward your push-up warrior goals. But if, like me, you love having a plan alongside your goals, here's a push-up progression to add into your training. (And guess what? None of the variations that I included in the progression are on your knees!) Add these exercises as workout finishers or on days you just want some extra movement in your routine. You don't have to do them every single day and can simply use them to check in with yourself once or twice a week during your strength training. (But feel free to add them into your daily morning routine!) Start at the level where you feel most comfortable, and move up at your own pace. There's no time limit to how long you remain at one level. If you're completing the level for the full amount of sets/reps, consider trying the following level next time. No matter what, just keep showing up, and you'll continue to surprise yourself.

Push-Up Form Reminders

- Hands—shoulder-width apart, in line with your sternum, placed directly below your shoulders (a wider placement will focus on your chest while a narrower placement will focus on your triceps)
- Elbows—slightly tucked, at a forty-five-degree angle from your body
- Shoulders—squeeze your shoulder blades together on the way down, drive them apart on the way up
- Head—neutral, avoid bending at your neck to reach for the ground with your face
- Core/glutes/quads—engaged and activated; you should feel your core contracting on the way up
- Chest—aim for between your hands; you should feel your chest stretching on the way down and contracting on the way back up
- Hips—slightly tucked in to prevent your lower back from sagging (squeeze those glutes!)
- Feet and/or knees—shoulder-width apart (a wider placement will add more stability if needed, but try not to lose focus of your overall form)
- Eyes—looking slightly forward instead of back toward your toes

Pro tip: To make sure that you have the proper form, visualize a broom resting all the way across your back touching three spots throughout your entire push-up: back of your head, your upper back, and your tailbone.

FOUR-LEVEL PUSH-UP PROGRESSION

Each level in the progression includes four exercises with three sets each. Each level of the progression begins with a plank hold, followed with eccentric push-ups, standard push-ups, and a final plank-hold variation. Level 1 begins with standing, using a wall to mimic the ground, and each level thereafter brings you closer down to the ground. Once you feel more comfortable at Level 4, replace the resistance-band-assisted push-ups with standard push-ups on your toes. If you're still struggling to complete one rep, it's okay! Try a standard push-up outside the progression when your body is warm, but not exhausted. If you're still tempted to drop to your knees, continue Level 4 a little longer until you're ready to give it a try again.

1. **Wall/Standing**
   - High-Plank (hold half-way down), *3 drop sets of 30/20/10 seconds*
   - Eccentric Push-Ups (Full Reset), *3 sets of 5 reps*
   - Push-Ups, *3 sets of 5 reps*
   - One-Arm Plank Hold, *3 sets of 10 seconds/arm*

2. **Counter/Incline**
   - High-Plank Hold, *3 drop sets of 30/20/10 seconds*
   - Eccentric Push-Ups (Full Reset), *3 sets of 5 reps*
   - Push-Ups, *3 sets of 5 reps*
   - Wide-Grip Plank Hold, *3 sets of 10 seconds*

3. **Bench*/Incline**
   ***Bench, sofa, chair, anything a little lower to the ground than a counter**
   - High-Plank Hold, *3 drop sets of 30/20/10 seconds*
   - Eccentric Push-Ups (Full Reset), *3 sets of 5 reps*
   - Push-Ups, *3 sets of 5 reps*
   - Decline High Plank, *3 sets of 10 seconds*

4. **Ground/Plank**
   - High-Plank Hold, *3 drop sets of 30/20/10 seconds*
   - Eccentric Push-Ups (Full Reset), *3 sets of 5 reps*
   - Resistance-Band-Assisted Push-Ups, *3 sets of 5 reps*
   - Diamond High-Plank Hold, *3 sets of 10 seconds*

Plank hold: Place your hands shoulder-width apart, palms flat on the surface (or the widest part of your palm on the corner of the surface if using an incline), feet hip-width apart, and shoulders directly above your wrists.

- *One-arm (Level 1) /* Place one hand either behind your back or at your side. Place the other hand against the wall more toward the center of your body, keeping your elbow slightly bent.
- *Wide-grip (Level 2) /* Place your hands slightly wider than shoulder width, keeping your elbows slightly bent.
- *Decline (Level 3) /* Similar position as a high-plank hold, with both of your feet propped up on a bench.
- *Diamond (Level 4) /* Place your hands together directly under your sternum, with the tips of your index fingers and thumbs touching, creating a diamond or triangle shape.

Eccentric push-up (full reset): Slowly lower your body (aim for a full four to five seconds). If pushing against a wall or counter, reset by stepping one foot forward once you reach the bottom and reset to a high-plank position. If pushing on an incline against a bench, reset by gently dropping your knees to the ground once you reach the bottom and reset to a high plank position. If pushing against the ground, reset by allowing your body to rest on the ground once you reach the bottom to lift yourself back up to a high-plank position. This exercise allows you to focus on the descending portion of the push-up in a slow and controlled manner.

ALL ABOUT SUPPLEMENTS AND GEAR

I'm often asked for recommendations about workout-related stuff like supplements and protein and leggings and knee sleeves. But before I dive in, an important caveat: these are all things that have worked for me. Everyone and every body is different, and what has helped me might not work for you. Remain open to options outside of these suggestions, especially if they are better for you and your body!

And do you need all of these things? Nope! Ignore toxic fitness culture's mainstream message of "one size fits all" for all the things you need to do all the things you love. It's always going to be up to you how much you invest in the gear and supplements that you use throughout your fitness journey. It's important to remember this and do a little extra research on the "life-changing health and wellness product promising x amount of weight lost in ten days" that keeps popping up in your sponsored ads before you consider buying it. Our weight-obsessed culture has a way of using misleading claims to hook as many women as possible into believing that certain ingredients will cure a bad body image. It's ridiculous, but it's always something to be aware of when choosing supplements and using gear to help you improve your athleticism.

Pre-Workout

I've always loved drinking a pre-workout supplement before any form of exercise. Something about the tingle wakes me right up and gives me the boost of energy for performance during a workout that I need every single time. Something to keep in mind when choosing a pre-workout drink is the amount of sugar and caffeine. If you are sensitive to caffeine, try avoiding drinks with a high dose (some have up to 500 mg of caffeine!) or ones that contain more natural caffeine. (For comparison, one cup of coffee is around 95 mg of caffeine.)[23] If you're not sure how your body will tolerate it, start with small amounts of a caffeinated pre-workout drink and slowly increase it to see how you tolerate it. The same goes for sugar. I usually avoid pre-workout drinks packed with sugar since they more times than not will make me crash and even negatively impact my workout by causing fatigue. Pre-workout supplements may increase your exercise capacity, but they are certainly not required to achieve a good workout. Like everything else, it's totally up to you.

I drink a pre-workout supplement thirty minutes before every workout and am ready to go by the time the workout starts. I make sure I always eat something light an hour before working out as well to avoid an upset stomach. Usually a light protein shake an hour before and a pre-workout drink thirty minutes before does just the trick to keep me full and not make me nauseous during my workout. If you're not sure what will work for you, always start with small portions and document how they make you feel. It might take some experimenting to find your sweet spot or if you should eat and/or drink pre-workout at all.

My personal faves: C4 and Universal Nutrition

Protein Powder

Protein shakes (and other fun things I make with protein powder sometimes) have definitely made a difference for me in increased strength and performance. Protein plays a major part in the building and repairing of muscles and tissues in our bodies, not to mention it's important for our hair, skin, blood, organs, antibodies, enzymes, and other body parts. It's the main building block of our body. You don't necessarily need to drink a bunch of protein shakes every day to get enough protein for your body. Just eating more of everyday foods that contain protein can be as beneficial. Animal protein is great if it's an option for you, but there are also plenty of vegetarian and vegan options as well. (For example: tofu, edamame, lentils, chickpeas, beans, quinoa, oats, nuts, etc.) Not everyone needs to supplement with extra protein, but it can certainly be useful for athletes (such as you and me!) because a higher protein intake will help build muscle and strength.

Before grabbing a giant tub of protein powder at your local nutrition shop for the first time, consider if you need to supplement with it at all. The National Academy of Medicine recommends 0.8 grams of protein per kilogram of body weight. To figure out how much that might be for you, multiply your body weight in pounds by 0.36, and that's how many grams of protein you need to meet your basic nutritional requirements. Take a moment to assess your current protein intake and see if it meets or already exceeds that requirement. Other factors that play a part in how much protein would be best for your body are your age, gender, and activity level. It's going to be different for everyone, even for those at the same exact weight, but using that simple equation can give you an idea if supplementing with protein powder might be helpful for you.[24]

On workout days, I drink two to three protein shakes that have 25 grams of protein each. Usually one in the morning with breakfast, one an hour before working out (or another type of protein snack on hand instead), and another thirty minutes to an hour after working out. On days I'm not working out, I usually stick to one protein shake or protein-packed snack that day in addition to regular meals that all include protein.

My personal faves: Dymatize and Universal Nutrition

Other Ideas and Ways to Incorporate Protein

- Use protein powder in pancakes, muffins, waffles, and any other yummy snacks.
- Include eggs with breakfast more often. One of my favorite things to do, which I learned from my trainer, is to mix eight ounces of egg whites with eight ounces of chocolate milk for a snack. I know it sounds wild but it doesn't taste anything like eggs!
- Add seeds or nuts on top of any of your side dishes.
- Include more lean meats in your meals, if you enjoy meat.
- If you're going to eat a salad, make it protein-rich with things like chicken, tuna, beans, or chickpeas.
- Put a little peanut butter on your fruit.

Remember that you don't have to count and track every gram of protein every day of your life in order to enjoy your fitness journey.

Creatine/Beta-Alanine

Some pre-workout supplements might already contain creatine and beta-alanine (the ingredient behind the tingle you feel from certain pre-workout drinks). I prefer to take creatine separately from my other pre-workout supplements. Creatine is a natural ingredient used to boost athletic performance and strength. It's safe to use and is one of the most effective supplements for building muscle and strength. Beta-alanine is a nonessential amino acid used by your body to produce carnosine, which helps improve your performance by reducing fatigue and increasing endurance. These supplements are not just for men—women benefit from taking them just as much.[25]

I mix 5 grams of creatine into my water bottle and drink it during my workouts. If I'm not working out that day, I'll drink it in the middle of the day and also mix in 3 grams of beta-alanine. Neither has any sort of taste, so you could mix them into anything. If I'm drinking a Gatorade during a workout, I'll mix it into that.

My personal faves: Universal Nutrition and ALLMAX Nutrition

Powerlifting Gear

A few lifting accessories have really made a difference for my powerlifting gains. (Yes, I call them gains, and it's quite liberating every time that I do.) They aren't necessary for everyone, but are definitely things to consider if you're planning on going after some personal records on squats and dead lifts.

- **Belts** are basically a tight harness that goes around your waist during a lift, creating abdominal pressure to support your spine. They are usually made out of neoprene, nylon, or leather and fasten with either a buckle, Velcro, or a quick-release lever (my personal favorite because it's easy to take off). If you're planning on introducing a belt to your heavier squats and dead lifts, make sure you're lifting with proper form beforehand to get the full benefits. I usually wear a belt for heavy squats, bench presses, and dead lifts (80 percent of my 1-rep max), as well as during any kind of barbell overhead-press exercises.

My personal fave: Inzer Forever Lever Belt 13mm (sizing up to 5X)

- **Wrist wraps** are two heavy-duty straps, usually made out of a blend of stretchy fabrics. Most are about a foot long and wrap around your wrists with Velcro. Their purpose is to keep your wrists from bending too far forward or backward and to lessen the pressure on your joints. I love wearing wrist wraps anytime I am lifting overhead, squatting, bench-pressing, or anything that is putting strain on my wrists and/or forearms.

   My personal fave: Inzer

- **Knee sleeves** compress and stabilize your knees during squats. They don't necessarily make you stronger or fix your form/technique, but chances are that they will improve any knee discomfort or pain. I mostly use them for heavy squats if I want extra support around my knees.

   My personal faves: StrongHouse Project (sizing up to 4X) and SBD (sizing up to 5X)

- **Lifters** are solid workout shoes with a slightly lifted heel that are used for squatting. Are they necessary? No. Are they beneficial? Absolutely. Most barbell lifts require your weight to remain on your heels, and the lifted heels of these shoes help make that happen, allowing you to maintain proper form.

   My personal fave: Nike Romaleos

- **Solid workout shoes.** It's important to choose a supportive shoe that fits the specific type of physical activity you're doing. Cross-trainers are great for dynamic moves in all directions, such as HIIT (High Intensity Interval Training) workouts and boot camps. A more flexible and cushioned sole option that helps to absorb impact would be better if you enjoy running.

And strength training shoes should have more stability with a flatter sole. You don't necessarily need a different type of shoe for every single physical activity, but taking a closer look at the shoes you wear when you're on the move might help prevent injury and allow you to perform at your best.

My personal fave: Under Armour TriBase Reign training shoes

You have a choice whether to invest in any supplements or weight-lifting gear. It's completely up to you, and there's no right or wrong way to embrace your fitness journey. With or without any of it, you're killing it just as you are.

EMBRACE YOUR INNER ATHLETE

My hands and knees trembled as I stepped into the Under Armour headquarters in Baltimore for the first time in early 2020 for their annual Human Performance Summit. Because I had stepped in as an athlete. As I glanced around the room and shook the hands of athletes from around the world, I noticed that my body was the largest there. Taking note of that, my entire nervous system instantly became overwhelmed with fear, doubt, and anxiety. I was panicking. I immediately questioned why I was invited when I was clearly the only athlete even remotely close to my size. My first instinct was to count myself out. I even considered skipping all of the workouts purely out of fear of embarrassing myself by not being able to do every move with precision and perfect form. But after succumbing to those moments of inner doubt, I knew that I couldn't let that fear get the best of me. I was there to prove that athletes come in all shapes and sizes. I imagined what it would look like if I nailed every single physical move throughout my time there. In workouts. In conversation. In my sheer presence. I knew that I needed to try.

An hour after I checked in, I was scheduled to take my personal fitness assessment. On my way over, I met another athlete. I nervously introduced myself and overexplained my philosophy and mind-set. To my surprise and relief, she listened intently and embraced everything I had to say. I'm not sure she even realized how much the conversation meant to me, as it gave me enough confidence to follow through with my assessment. As part of the assessment, I was asked to execute five push-ups. Before I could get all the way down on the ground to begin, it was mentioned it was okay to modify them if I'd prefer. I smiled and did five perfect push-ups on my toes. It was the first time I got a double take. And it felt good.

Later that evening, representatives from Under Armour provided all the attending athletes with a welcome party on the rooftop of our hotel. I sat on a couch in a corner by myself for an hour before deciding to make my way back down to my room, order room service, and call it a night. I was terrified of the next four days, even after my personal fitness assessment went well, and needed some downtime.

Once I made it back to my room, I popped my earbuds in and sat down, staring out the floor-to-ceiling window that overlooked a beautiful Baltimore skyline. The Under Armour sign was lit up bright and clear, marking where I would be completing my first workout, a boxing class, the next morning. Doubt started to plague me, as I had never taken a boxing class before. Suddenly, I was crying, tears pouring down my face as I sobbed for what felt like the length of an entire Taylor Swift album. I had felt fear before in my lifetime, but nothing was quite close to this. As my tears began to slow and my breathing returned to normal, I stood up and placed both hands on the window. I knew that I needed to talk myself out of this doubt.

So, I thought about the time I competed in CG Games (and completed every single event) at eight months postpartum. I thought about how it was so hard and yet so worth it to witness my athletic ability. I remembered competing in my first dead-lift competition, crushing my personal record. It was terrifying and yet so worth it. I remembered competing in my first full powerlifting meet, winning first place. It was so overwhelming and yet so valuable training for something I had no idea I could win. I recalled competing in my first combine, ranking in my age category for a good portion of the day, seeing my name up on the big screen. It was exhausting and yet worth the bloody hands when I heard the event timer shout, "Eighty-three reps!," as my body hit the ground. Remembering these incredible moments helped me regain my focus.

The next morning, I showed up for the boxing class and gave that shit my all. I introduced myself to those around me, making lifelong friends. When getting sneak peeks at the forthcoming the women's apparel line, I got uncomfortable and asked questions about sizing and inclusivity. And I stood tall in my five-foot-three-inch body that was so different from every other body in the room. I had arrived. I continued to show up throughout that week, fully engaged and confident in the yoga class, the lessons, the dinners, the panels, the recovery sessions, the workouts, and everything else Under Armour had to offer. I had realized that I won't always feel ready, but it will always be worth trying.

And I felt happy. I felt happy in a body that I had assumed only deserved anything but joy. I laughed and I cried and I felt thankful—thankful for a body society had told me wasn't supposed to embrace athleticism over weight loss. This summit wasn't my first time on this emotional roller coaster and it wasn't going to be the last, but I still showed up. My body was always ready. I just needed to be reminded to give it a chance for once. And I'm so fucking glad that I did.

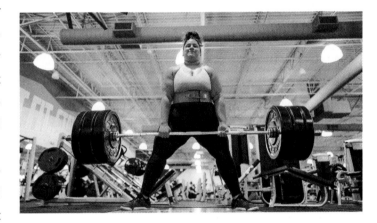

So, as you ride this emotional roller coaster of life and fitness, remember that it's not one swift moment that will get you from doubt to transformation. It won't happen in the completion of a certain number of events, or in an increase in your athleticism, or in the perfection of every powerlift or fitness assessment. Your journey is not in the breakdowns or the breakthroughs. It has simply (and always been) inside you, the athlete. So, I hope you never forget to unapologetically embrace every hard-as-hell moment. Even when that shit gets tough because, trust me, you are tougher. Remember that is how it begins. So, say it proud and say it out loud: *"I am an athlete, too."* I believe you. I see you. Now, do you believe and see it, too?

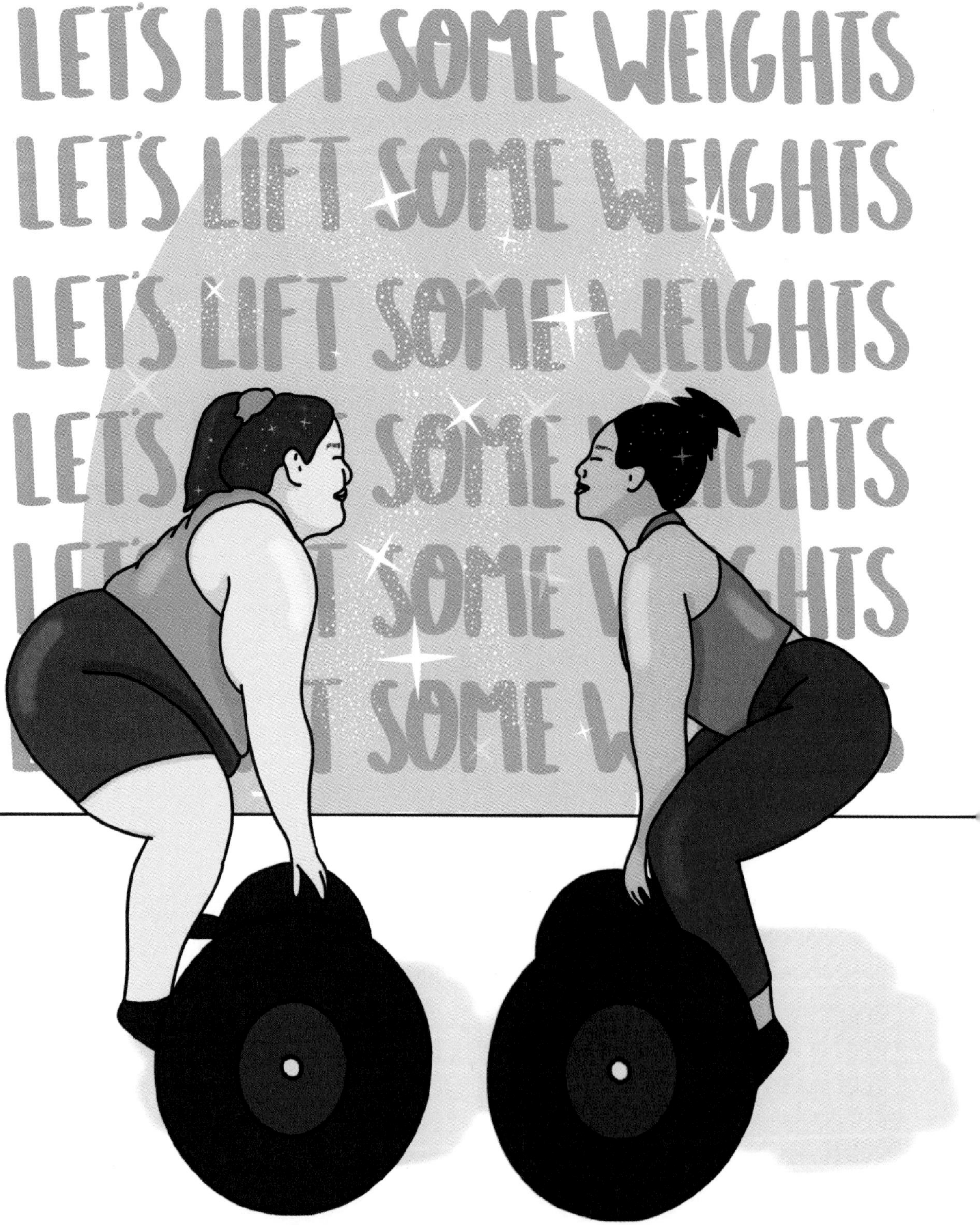
LET'S LIFT SOME WEIGHTS
LET'S LIFT SOME WEIGHTS
LET'S LIFT SOME WEIGHTS

PART 5

The Part Where We Pick Up Some Weights

ABOUT THE GUIDE

The Twelve-Week Strength Training Guide that follows is based on a push-pull-legs training method that is similar to how I train. Essentially, I've separated most of the push muscle exercises (chest, shoulders, triceps) and pull muscle exercises (back, biceps) by placing them on different days. I also separated an entire day for legs, which will occur at the end of each week. Below are three workouts for each week, with a rest day in between each workout. Every two weeks, for a little extra recovery, I've included a Self-Care Day that falls on an extended three-day rest period. I listed several examples of what self-care could look like for you, but it's also totally up to you how you choose to recover and take care of your body. All of the workouts require minimal equipment and can all be done at home. If you're planning on following my powerlifting version of the guide (page 165), you'll also need access to a gym to use barbells if you don't have those at home. If you're new to strength training, I suggest starting with the strength-training guide for one full round before transitioning some of the exercises to powerlifts, unless you are working with a trainer and/or experienced partner to spot you and assist with your form. The example calendar is also completely customizable, but I do encourage you to stick with three workouts per week in their order, if possible, for the best strength results. And no matter what, be sure to rest and recover as needed!

WARMING UP AND COOLING DOWN
ALL THE GOODS

Pro tip: Create a separate music playlist for your warm-up and cool-down routines to keep you motivated for them. Having a whole separate music vibe for pre- and postworkout stretches / foam rolling has been a game changer for me! You can follow me on Spotify and check out all of my playlists with my favorite music for workouts, warming up, and just feeling all kinds of empowered on any given day.

Warm-Up

A five-minute warm-up routine is usually ideal for most people, and I highly recommend it before every strength-training workout. I can't even tell you how many times I just didn't care much about anything other than the workout and found myself struggling not only to get the most benefit out of my workouts, but also to maximize my range of motion, much less be able to maintain good form and prevent injury. (I lost count in the beginning of my lifting journey of my minor injuries here and there during the time I was avoiding these kinds of extra moments with my body). I was stubborn about it for a long time and finally started trying warm-ups prior to a workout, and let me just say—warm up! Seriously, it makes a difference. Adding a warm-up filled with dynamic stretches/moves is perfect if you want to increase your mobility (helping your joints move through a full range of motions without any discomfort) and get your blood pumping. My mobility has improved since fully engaging in warm-ups, which only increased my range of motion. It doesn't take much to warm up your muscles and joints in preparation for an awesome sweat celebration. Your body will thank you for it.

I like to warm up by doing a few dynamic stretches such as Toy Soldiers, Inchworms, and Overhead Body Squats. I'll pair that with a few sets of light cardio movements such as Jumping Jacks, Butt Kicks, or High Knees. After this five-minute warm-up, I continue warming up just a bit more by focusing on the specific movements and muscles that I'll be using during that workout. For example, if the first set of the workout is weighted squats, I'll do a warm-up set without weights, using my body weight only. If the weight per set is a bit heavier (less reps per set), I'll add in a second warm-up set of half the weight. By the time I begin my first set, my body is warm and going to benefit from what I'll be focusing on throughout the rest of my workout. And it only takes five to ten minutes, which goes by quickly if you have some good jams playing to pump you up!

Here's one of my favorite ways to get warmed up for all of my strength-training workouts!

Dynamic Five-Minute Warm-Up

- Marching High Knees *(30 seconds)*
- Overhead Body Squats *(10 total)*
- Butt Kicks *(30 seconds)*
- Toy Soldiers *(10 per leg)*
- Torso Twists *(30 seconds)*
- Inchworms *(5 total)*
- Arm Up-and-Downs *(30 seconds)*
- Jumping Jacks *(20 total)*

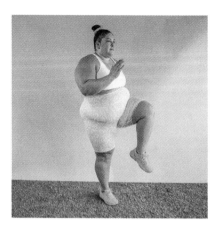

Marching High Knees: Lift your knees up one at a time, marching in place. Try to stand tall and relax your shoulders while engaging your core.

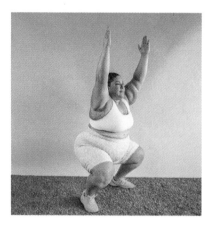

Overhead Body Squats: Stand with your feet shoulder-width apart and your toes slightly turned outward. Hold both arms up above your head, engage your core while hinging at the hips first, then bend your knees while lowering into a squat position where your thighs are either parallel or below parallel with the floor. Exhale and press heels into the ground to stand. This is one rep. Keep both arms up above your head the entire time. (Modification: Squat down into a chair. Use another chair or table to assist, if needed, as you press your heels into the ground to stand.)

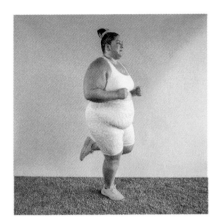

Butt Kicks: Stand with your feet hip-width apart. Kick back your right heel toward your butt by contracting your hamstring muscle, alternating your heels at a steady pace that feels comfortable for you.

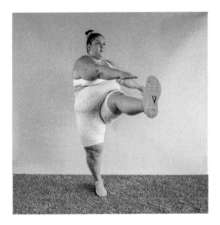

Toy Soldiers: Keeping your legs straight, try to kick one of your legs out while your opposite hand swings forward to reach for your toes. Try not to overextend. You can do this in a stationary position or walking forward. (Modification: Hold on to a chair or table as you kick your legs out. Kick the leg on the same side as the hand with which you're holding the chair, in order to reach for your toes with the opposite hand. It's okay if you can't reach them yet. Reach for your knee or shin, whichever is currently in reach.)

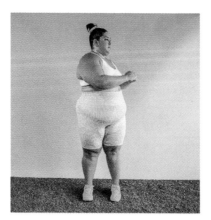

Torso Twists: Stand with your feet hip-width apart. Rotate your torso from one side to the other, while keeping your pelvis facing forward.

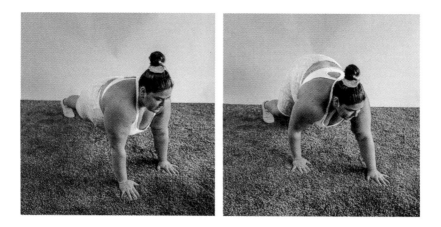

Inchworms: Start in a standing position with your feet hip-width apart. Hinge forward at your hips until your hands are placed down on the floor and begin walking your hands forward into a high-plank position. Once in this position, your shoulders should be directly above your wrists. Walk your hands back toward your feet and stand up. This is 1 rep. (Modification: Once your hands are placed down on the floor, walk your hands out forward to a downward-dog position before walking your hands back toward your feet and standing up.)

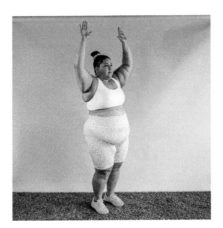

Arm Up-and-Downs: Standing up straight with your feet hip-width apart and your arms by your sides, swing both arms up above your head (like you're about to go down a roller coaster!). Then swing them both back down by your sides.

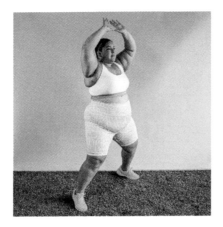

Jumping Jacks: Standing straight up with your feet hip-width apart, knees slightly bent, and arms by your sides, jump both of your feet out to the sides while at the same time raising your arms up above your head. From this position, jump both of your feet back to their starting position while bringing your arms back down to your sides. This is 1 rep. (Modification: Instead of jumping both feet out to the sides at the same time, step out one foot to the side while raising both arms up above your head. Then repeat with the other leg.)

Cooldown

The workout is done, and you're glowing! Yeah! But before you jump in the shower to celebrate your hard work, maybe try finishing with a light cooldown if you can. While we focused more on dynamic stretches during the warm-up, the cooldown will include more static stretching, meaning we hold stretches for twenty to thirty seconds. Just like the warm-up, I neglected these exercises for far too long before realizing how beneficial a proper cooldown can be. Stretching postworkout will help relieve all of that muscle tension that you built up during your workout and will help reduce your soreness. I know, warming up and cooling down just aren't as exciting as the main workout, and it can be hard to give your body a few more minutes of movement. But trust me, adding on a few stretches to the end of your workout will feel so good! It doesn't have to be long or complicated—a simple five minutes can make a difference! I'm just a big fan of a real good postworkout stretch and what it has done for me and my body! But as with everything else in this chapter, do what feels right for you.

Give this cooldown a try after your next workout and check in with yourself to see how you feel. Listen to your body and stretch anything that feels like it needs a good stretching!

Five-Move Full-Body Cooldown

- Cat-Cow *(30 seconds total)*
- Runner's Lunge *(30 seconds on each side)*
- Pigeon Pose *(30 seconds on each side)*
- Scorpion *(30 seconds on each side)*
- Child's Pose *(30 seconds total)*

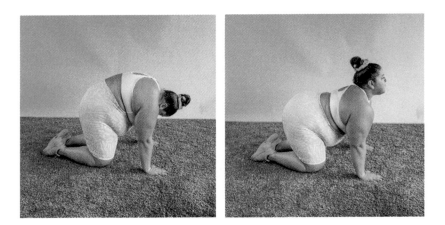

Cat-Cow: Start with your hands and knees on the floor. Your knees should be under your hips with your wrists under your shoulders. From a neutral spine position, with an engaged core and a flat back, take a deep breath. When you exhale, round your spine toward the ceiling as if your belly button is being pulled up. At the same time, tuck your chin in toward your chest. (This is the cat shape.) As you inhale, slowly arch your back down while allowing your stomach to be completely relaxed and tilt your head back while pulling your tailbone toward the ceiling. (This is the cow shape.) Move slowly back and forth for thirty seconds, inhaling in the cow pose and exhaling in the cat pose.

This is also a great stretch to do first thing in the morning!

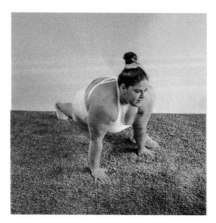

Runner's Lunge: Start with your hands and knees flat on the floor. Bring your right foot up to just outside your right hand, or as close to it as possible. You can either raise your left knee up off the ground as you hold this stretch, or keep your knee placed on the ground. Lean forward for a few seconds at a time to feel the stretch in your hip, shifting your weight forward and back for thirty seconds before switching to the other side.

Another optional add-on is to leave your left hand placed on the ground while twisting your torso to the right and reaching up to the ceiling with your right hand. Do the same on the other side.

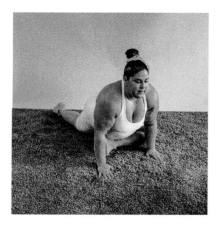

Pigeon Pose: Start with your hands and knees on the floor. Bring your right knee up just below your right hand and your right foot up just below your left hand. Your right shin should now be resting on the floor. The farther forward you place your right heel, the deeper the stretch will be. But you can keep your knee bent only as much as feels comfortable, especially if you're a beginner. Slide your left leg back behind you with the front of your thigh on the floor. The top of your left foot should be flat on the ground. Try to lower your right hip to the floor while walking your hands forward and laying your torso down over your right leg. Inhale and exhale deeply as you hold this pose for thirty seconds, then slowly walk your hands back to an upright position. Switch sides.

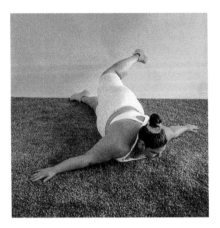

Scorpion: Lie on your stomach with your chest flat on the ground. Make a T-shape on the ground with your arms. Lift your right foot off the ground and cross it over to your left side reaching as far as you can while keeping your T shape and chest flat on the ground. Hold this for thirty seconds, then switch sides.

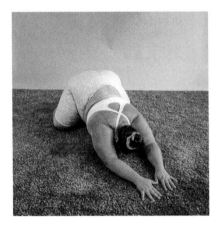

Child's Pose: Sit on your heels, open up your knees, and lean all the way forward on the ground in the space between your legs. Stretch your arms out in front of you with your palms flat on the ground. Relax your forehead on the ground and release all of the tension in your body. Hold this pose for thirty seconds. Or however long you need!

An optional add-on is to take your right arm and reach it underneath your left arm onto the ground with your palm facing the ceiling and right shoulder/arm pressed into the ground. Do the same on the other side.

FOAM ROLLING

I know it can feel like foam rolling is reserved only for the most elite athletes, but it's a routine worth trying, no matter your fitness level. If you're moving your body and being active, you'll definitely benefit in some way from foam rolling, even if it's not on a regular schedule. If you've ever foam rolled before, you know it's a bit harder to commit to it since it isn't quite the most, well, um, comfortable thing to do. But don't worry, pushing through that little bit of discomfort will release any tightness and tension that has built up in your muscles after they've been worked hard.

How does it work?

Foam rolling is a self-massage using continuous pressure on your muscles to loosen them up by use of a foam roller (those tube-shaped things people lie on and roll all over). Releasing all of this tension in your muscles will likely decrease any discomfort, allow you to move around a bit more easily, and help increase your mobility. Think of it as another form of stretching; whether that's during your warm-up or cooldown (or even on a rest day) is totally up to you.

My Five Foam-Rolling Tips

1. **Roll slowly over targeted muscle areas, avoiding tendons, bones, your lower back, and any injured areas.** Spend around twenty to thirty seconds rocking back and forth slowly on one targeted muscle at a time, slowing down in areas feeling extratight. You're rolling over all of that tight fascia (the connective tissue that surrounds your bones, muscles, and joints). You may have

heard someone describe muscle tightness as "knots." Once you finish in one area, move on to the next part of your body until you've rolled all areas that you want to target.

2. **Start by placing the foam roller toward the center of your body on the meaty part of your targeted muscle, slowly rolling away from that center.** For example, when rolling out your hamstrings, start around the top of your hamstring just underneath your butt (that meaty part of your hamstring) and slowly roll away until you get to the top of the back of your knee. Then slowly roll back up to the starting position.

3. **Keep your muscles relaxed and avoid flexing.** Foam rolling can feel a bit uncomfortable, especially if you're extratight, and it's natural to tense up during it. But try to stay as relaxed as possible, as being overly tense will potentially prevent the foam roller from targeting those deep tissues.

4. **Foam roll either before or after working out—whichever works for you.** If you're foam rolling before working out, try quicker and a bit lighter strokes to get your blood flowing in your muscles. If you're foam rolling after working out, try longer and deeper strokes to lighten up the tension in your muscles. You could even do this on any random day, whether you're working out or not. It will be just as beneficial for your body in recovery. It's also a great addition to your before-bed routine if you're like me and love having an end-of-day wind-down routine.

5. **If you're new to foam rolling, try a low- to medium-density foam roller.** They also come in all different sizes, but an eighteen-inch or twenty-four-inch one can usually target most parts of your body. You can find a perfect, basic foam roller for around $15 at plenty of online retailers. You can always get fancier later with higher densities and extra textures if you feel ready to explore those.

Try a few of these foam-rolling moves after your next workout and see if any of them make a difference for you! I love adding a few of these after a tough workout before my cooldown. I usually pick moves that will target the muscles I just got done working, such as focusing on lower-body moves after leg day and upper-body moves after chest or back day. You aren't required to stretch and foam roll before and after every workout to benefit from moving your body however you're choosing to move it. But I want to remind you that foam rolling isn't reserved for the most elite athletes. We all have bodies, and they all deserve to be given a little extra love every now and then. It's totally up to you how you choose to give it to yours. No matter what you choose, I hope you know that you've always deserved it.

Lower-Body Foam-Rolling Moves

- **Quads:** Lie facedown on your stomach with the foam roller under your upper thigh, near your hip on the meaty part of your thigh (not on your hip bone or joint). You can open up your other leg/hip to allow the inside of that knee to rest on the floor if that's more comfortable. Place your elbows and forearms on the ground to help stabilize and balance your weight on the foam roller. Roll two to three inches down your thigh, then back up your thigh slowly. Continue for twenty to thirty seconds and repeat on the other leg.

- **Hamstrings:** Sit on the ground with your legs extended. Place the foam roller underneath your thighs near your glutes, lifting your body up to allow your weight to rest on the foam roller. Slowly roll down over your hamstrings and just above the back of your knees. It might feel more comfortable to roll one leg at a time. If so, place the other leg on the ground to help hold your body up. Continue for twenty to thirty seconds.

- **Hip flexors:** Lie directly on the ground, on your right side. Place the foam roller underneath your pelvic bone at the very top of your thigh. Place your right elbow and forearm on the ground while using your left leg to balance and help hold your body up. Roll from your pelvic bone to your hip bone, move slowly back and forth about one to two inches, and rotate your pelvis toward the floor and away from it as you roll. Continue for twenty to thirty seconds before switching to the left side.

- **Glutes:** Sit on top of the foam roller while on the floor, placing it in the middle of your glutes. Cross your right ankle over your left knee. Lean toward your right leg to get deeper into your glute muscle. Use your left leg, which is placed on the ground, to help roll back and forth for twenty to thirty seconds before switching sides.
- **Calves:** Sit on the floor and place the foam roller under one of your calves (on the meaty center) with your hands flat on the ground and the other leg flat on the ground for support. Lift your hips off the floor and roll the bottom half of your calf up and down, stopping about an inch or two above your Achilles tendon. Gently rotate your leg side to side and continue rolling the lower half of your calf for twenty to thirty seconds. Repeat on the upper part of your calf, then switch legs.

Upper-Body Foam-Rolling Moves

- **Upper back:** Position the foam roller underneath your upper back, just below your shoulder blades, and lie on your back. Keep your feet flat on the floor with your arms either down by your side or crossed on top of your chest. Lightly engage your core and lift your lower body up into a bridge position. Hold this for a few seconds before shifting your hips down toward your heels about two to three inches, allowing the foam roller to slowly move up your back (stop at the top of your shoulder blades, just before your neck). Continue for twenty to thirty seconds.
- **Lats:** Lie on your right side, keeping your right hip on the ground, and place the foam roller horizontally under your armpit with your right arm extended overhead and against the floor. Your left hand and left leg can be placed on the floor out in front of you (on the floor or on the foam roller) for support and to help guide the movement of your body. Use your left leg to push your body upward to allow the foam roller to move downward against your lat. Pause once your foam roller reaches the bottom of your rib cage, then slowly roll it back up toward your armpit. Continue for twenty to thirty seconds before switching sides.

- **Shoulders/triceps:** Lie on your right side, keeping your right hip on the ground, and place the foam roller underneath your right shoulder up against your shoulder/deltoid. Your left arm can be placed on the floor out in front of you to help guide the movement of your body. Use your left leg to push your body upward to allow the foam roller to move downward against your shoulder. Pause once the foam roller reaches the bottom of your deltoid muscle toward the middle of your arm, then slowly roll back up toward the top of your shoulder. Lean and rotate your body slightly to hit your upper back and triceps as well. Continue for twenty to thirty seconds before switching sides.

- **Pecs:** Lie facedown and place the foam roller diagonally on the right side of your chest, closer to the center of your chest than your armpit. Extend your right arm up off the ground. Lift your hips off the ground, using your left hand and knees to brace yourself. Curl your toes under and slowly guide your body against the roller from just above your breast across the front of your armpit. Continue for twenty to thirty seconds before switching sides.

TWELVE-WEEK STRENGTH TRAINING GUIDE

	Sunday	Monday	Tuesday	Wednesday	Thursday	Friday	Saturday
Week 1		Chest A		Back A		Legs A	
Week 2	self-care		Chest B		Back B		Legs B
Week 3		Chest C		Back C		Legs C	
Week 4	self-care		Chest A (up weights)		Back A		Legs A
Week 5		Chest B		Back B		Legs B	
Week 6	self-care		Chest C		Back C		Legs C
Week 7		Chest A (up weights)		Back A		Legs A	
Week 8	self-care		Chest B		Back B		Legs B
Week 9		Chest C		Back C		Legs C	
Week 10	self-care		Chest A (up weights)		Back B		Legs B
Week 11		Chest B		Back B		Legs B	
Week 12	self-care		Chest C		Back C		Legs C

A WORKOUTS

Chest A

Five straight sets: Complete the first exercise for the full amount of sets before moving on to the next exercise. Rest as needed between sets and exercises, at least three to four minutes.

1. DB Chest Press *(5 sets, 10 reps)*
2. DB Overheard Press *(5 sets, 10 reps)*
3. DB Chest Flies *(3 sets, 15 reps)*
4. Single DB Chest Press *(3 sets, 15 reps)*
5. DB Triceps Kickbacks *(3 sets, 15 reps)*

Powerlift Option: Replace the Dumbbell Chest Press exercise with a Barbell Bench Press (see page 170).

Powerlift Option: Replace the Dumbbell Overhead Press with a Barbell Overhead Press (see page 175).

Dumbbell Chest Press

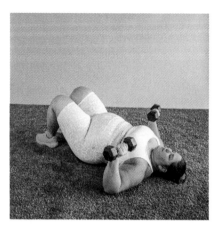

- Lie on your back with your knees bent and feet flat on the floor. Hold a dumbbell in each hand with your elbows out at an angle to your sides.
- Squeezing your shoulder blades together, push the dumbbells upward by extending your arms, straightening your elbows completely. Avoid bouncing the dumbbells together.
- Slowly bend your elbows to lower the dumbbells until your elbows are just above the floor. Pause for a second before pushing the weights back up for another rep. Avoid resting your arms on the ground between reps.

Modify Down
- Use lighter weights.
- Use a light resistance band instead of dumbbells.

Modify Up
- Raise to a hip bridge while pressing.
- Hover your feet above the ground a few inches while pressing.

Dumbbell Overhead Press

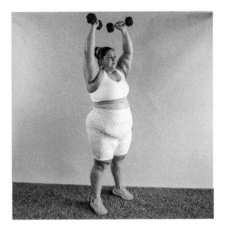

- Stand with your feet about hip-width apart. Hold a dumbbell in each hand and rest them at shoulder height, with your elbows bent and palms facing each other.
- Keeping your core engaged, press both dumbbells overhead, straightening your elbows completely.
- Slowly bend your elbows to lower the dumbbells back down to shoulder height.

Modify Down
- Use lighter weights, or one dumbbell with both hands.
- Sit instead of standing.
- Use a light resistance band instead of dumbbells.

Modify Up
- Add a squat between reps.

Dumbbell Chest Flies

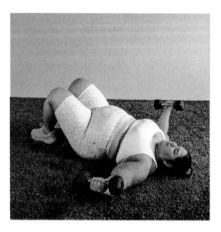

- Lie on your back with your knees bent and feet flat on the floor. Hold a dumbbell in each hand and press them together straight above your chest, with your elbows straight and palms facing each other.
- Keeping your core engaged, slowly separate and lower the dumbbells toward the floor while maintaining a soft roundness with your arms (as if you're hugging a tree), straight wrists, and lightly bent elbows.
- Slowly raise the dumbbells by squeezing your chest and maintaining the soft roundness in your arms. Avoid bouncing the dumbbells together.

Modify Down
- Use lighter weights.
- Use a light resistance band instead of dumbbells.

Modify Up
- Raise to a hip bridge while lifting.
- Hover your feet above the ground a few inches while lifting.

Single Dumbbell Chest Press

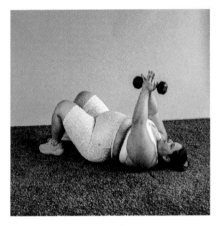

- Lie on your back with your knees bent and feet flat on the floor. Hold a single dumbbell between your palms just above your chest. Palms should be squeezing together just below the handle and fingers shouldn't be interlocked.
- Squeezing your chest, push the dumbbell upward by extending your arms, straightening your elbows completely. Pause and squeeze your chest at the top.
- Slowly bend your elbows to lower the dumbbell.

Modify Down

- Use a lighter weight. Alternatively, drop the dumbbell and place palms together.

Modify Up

- Raise to a hip bridge while pressing.
- Hover your feet above the ground a few inches while pressing.

Dumbbell Triceps Kickbacks

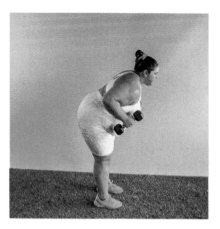

- Stand with your feet about hip-width apart. Hold a dumbbell in each hand at your side, with your palms facing each other. Hinge forward at your hips with your knees slightly bent.
- Engaging your core and keeping your back flat, straighten your elbows by pushing the dumbbells back.
- Control the weight as you bring it back to the starting position. Avoid swinging the dumbbells.

Modify Down
- Perform one arm at a time by supporting yourself with a chair or bench with one arm and executing the exercise with the other.

Modify Up
- Pause for one to two seconds at the top of the extension.

Back A

Three supersets: Complete the first and second exercises (1A and 1B) as one continuous set before resting and repeating for another set until all sets are complete. Then move on to the next superset (2A and 2B), followed by the final superset (3A and 3B). Rest as needed between sets and supersets, at least three to four minutes. Try not to pause for too long between A/B exercises.

1A. DB Renegade Rows *(5 sets, 5 reps/arm)*
1B. DB Preacher Curls *(5 sets, 5 reps/arm)*
2A. Superman Pull Downs *(4 sets, 10 reps)*
2B. Shoulder Taps *(4 sets, 10 reps)*
3A. DB Lat Pullovers *(3 sets, 12 reps)*
3B. Single DB Biceps Curls *(3 sets, 12 reps/arm)*

Powerlift Option: Begin the workout with Barbell Dead Lifts, then continue through the rest of the workout (see page 172).

Dumbbell Renegade Rows

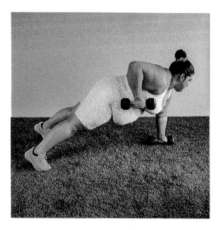

- In a high plank on the floor, hold a dumbbell in each hand, with your hands shoulder-width apart, feet hip-width apart, and shoulders directly above your wrists.
- Engaging your core and glutes, pull your right elbow back and lift the dumbbell toward the bottom of your chest. Keep your elbow close to your body. Avoid rocking by keeping your core and glutes engaged and tight.
- Lower the dumbbell back to the ground. Repeat with your left arm.

Modify Down

- Separate your feet farther apart (wider than hip-width) to help with stability.
- Instead of a high plank, drop down to your knees, keeping them wide for stability.
- Use lighter weights, or remove the dumbbells.

Modify Up

- Add a push-up between reps.

Dumbbell Preacher Curls

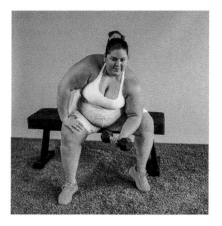

- Sitting on a bench and bent slightly forward, hold a dumbbell in your right hand and place your right elbow on the inside of your right knee with your elbow straight. Place your left hand on your left knee for stability.
- Slowly curl the dumbbell up with your palm facing your shoulder. Your elbow should remain pressed against your knee.
- Lower the dumbbell back down, controlling the weight and allowing some resistance. Repeat with your left arm.

Modify Down
- Use lighter weights.
- Use a light resistance band instead of dumbbells.

Modify Up
- Place a light resistance band under your feet and wrap around your dumbbell to create extra resistance as the weight is lifted.

Superman Pull Downs

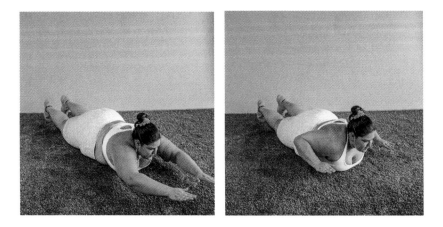

- Lie on your stomach with your arms extended above your head and palms facing down.
- Squeezing your glutes and lower back, raise your arms and the top of your chest up above the ground, creating a Y shape.
- Squeeze your back to pull your elbows toward the sides of your chest, pausing in this position for a moment before extending your arms back up to the starting position.

Modify Down
- Extend one arm at a time while bracing with the other arm.

Modify Up
- Lift your lower body off the ground during the entire exercise (Full Superman).
- Use a resistance band wrapped around a sturdy surface in front of you.

Shoulder Taps

- In a high plank on the floor, place your hands shoulder-width apart, palms flat on the floor, feet hip-width apart, and shoulders directly above your wrists.
- Engaging your core, lift your right hand up off the ground and tap your left shoulder. Place your hand back down on the ground and repeat with your left hand. Avoid rocking at your hips.
- Completing both sides = 1 rep.

Modify Down
- Separate feet farther apart (wider than hip-width) to help with stability.
- Instead of a high plank on the ground, use a higher incline such as a counter, bench, or sofa.

Modify Up
- When tapping your shoulder, pause for one to two seconds before placing your hand back down.

Dumbbell Lat Pullovers

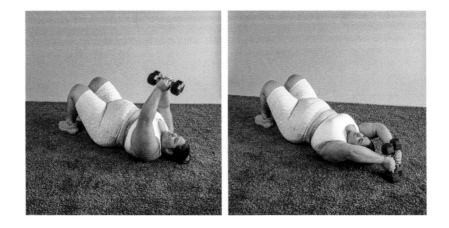

- Lie on your back with your knees bent and feet flat on the floor. Hold a dumbbell in each hand and extend out over your head on the ground, with your elbows straight and palms facing each other.
- Engaging your core and keeping your lower back pressed into the ground, slowly raise your arms until your dumbbells are above your chest. Your elbows should remain straight throughout.
- Slowly lower your arms back to their starting position above your head. Avoid bouncing off the ground.

Modify Down
- Use lighter weights (or one single dumbbell).
- Bend your elbows slightly.

Modify Up
- Raise to a hip bridge while pressing.
- Hover your feet above the ground a few inches while lifting.

Single Dumbbell Biceps Curls (see page 139)

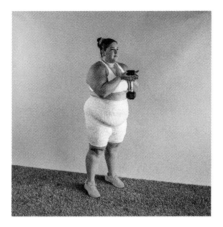

Legs A

Five straight sets: Complete the first exercise for the full amount of sets before moving on to the next exercise. Rest as needed between sets and exercises, at least three to four minutes.

1. DB Squats *(5 sets, 10 reps)*
2. DB Swings *(5 sets, 10 reps)*
3. DB Hip Thrusts *(3 sets, 15 reps)*
4. DB Hamstring Curls *(3 sets, 15 reps)*
5. DB Lateral Lunges *(3 sets, 15 reps)*

Powerlift Option: Replace the Dumbbell Squats exercise with a Barbell Back Squat (see page 167).

Dumbbell Squats

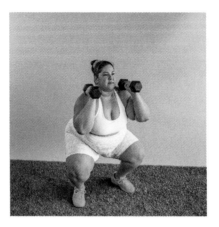

- Stand with your feet about shoulder-width apart and your toes slightly turned outward. Hold a dumbbell in each hand and rest them at shoulder height, with your elbows bent and palms facing each other.
- Engaging your core while hinging at the hips first, bend your knees while lowering into a squat position where your thighs are either parallel or below parallel with the floor.
- Exhale and press your heels into the ground to stand.

Modify Down

- Use lighter weights, or drop the dumbbells and do body-weight squats.
- Do a half squat, working your way down to a full squat as your strength and mobility begin to improve.
- Squat down into a chair.

Modify Up

- Use heavier weights.
- Lift one leg/foot behind you onto a chair or bench and do Bulgarian Split Squats.

Dumbbell Swings

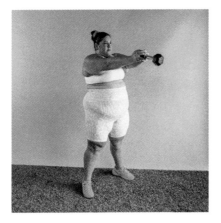

- Stand with your feet shoulder-width apart. Hold a dumbbell with one hand in front of the other at the center of the dumbbell.
- Bending your knees slightly and without rounding your lower back, push your hips back then hinge forward at your hips, placing the dumbbell between your legs.
- Squeeze your glutes and thrust your hips forward using the momentum (not your arms or shoulders) to swing the dumbbell up and forward to chest level. At the top of the movement, contract your core, glutes, and quads. Repeat.

Modify Down
- Use a lighter weight.

Modify Up
- Use a heavier weight or a kettlebell.

Dumbbell Hip Thrusts

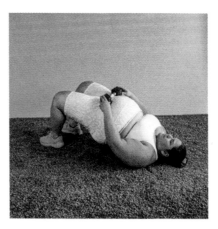

- Lie on your back with your knees bent, feet flat on the floor. Hold a dumbbell with both hands and rest it just below your hip bones.
- Engaging your core, push through your heels and lift your hips off the floor until they align with your knees. Squeeze your glutes at the top.
- Lower your hips back down, only lightly tapping the ground and keeping core engaged.

Modify Down
- Remove the dumbbell.

Modify Up
- Use a resistance band around your thighs, just above your knees.
- Lift one leg at a time, keeping it raised above the ground.

Dumbbell Hamstring Curls

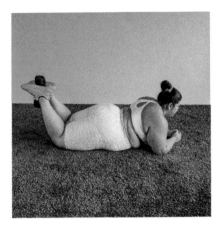

- Lie facedown on a bench. Place a dumbbell between your feet. (Test with a lighter weight to get the form right before using a heavier weight.)
- Contracting your hamstrings, bend your knees and curl the dumbbell up toward the ceiling.
- Slowly lower your feet back down until you feel a slight stretch in your hamstrings.

Modify Down
- Use a lighter weight.
- Lie on the floor instead of a bench.

Modify Up
- Work your way up to a heavier dumbbell. (Be sure to get comfortable with the form while using lighter weights beforehand.)

Dumbbell Lateral Lunges

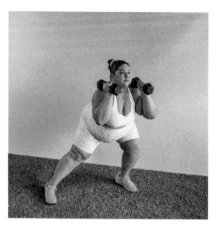

- Stand with your feet shoulder-width apart. Hold a dumbbell in each hand and rest them at shoulder height, with your elbows bent and palms facing each other.
- Engaging your core and keeping your feet parallel, step your right foot wide to the right without bending your left knee.
- Keeping your left leg straight, your back flat, and your chest up, bend your right knee, set your hips back, and lower your body until your right thigh is parallel to the floor. Push off your right foot to return to a standing position and repeat with the left leg.

Modify Down

- Drop the dumbbells and use your body weight only.
- Lower your hips halfway instead of all the way to knee level.

Modify Up

- Add two to three pulses at the bottom of each lunge.

B WORKOUTS

Chest B

Five straight sets: Complete the first exercise for the full amount of sets before moving on to the next exercise. Rest as needed between sets and exercises, at least three to four minutes.

1. Push-Ups *(5 drop sets, 5-4-3-2-1)*
2. Single DB Chest Press *(3 sets, 10 reps)*
3. Single DB Standing Arnold Press *(3 sets, 10/arm)*
4. Eccentric DB Hammer Curls *(3 sets, 5 reps—paused, slow on way down)*
5. Eccentric DB Lateral Raises *(3 sets, 5 reps—paused, slow on way down)*

Powerlift Option: Replace the Push-Ups exercise with a Barbell Bench Press (see page 170).

Powerlift Option: Replace the Standing Arnold Press with a Barbell Overhead Press (see page 175).

Push-Ups

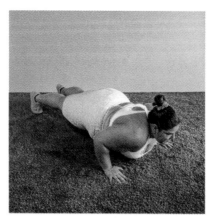

Start with 5 reps on the first set. Drop to 4 reps on the second set. Drop to 3 reps on the third set. Drop to 2 reps on the fourth set. Drop to 1 rep on the fifth set. (See page 80 for more on push-ups.)

Single Dumbbell Chest Press (see page 115)

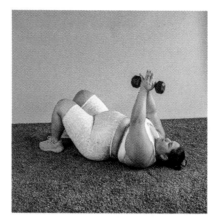

Single Dumbbell Standing Arnold Press

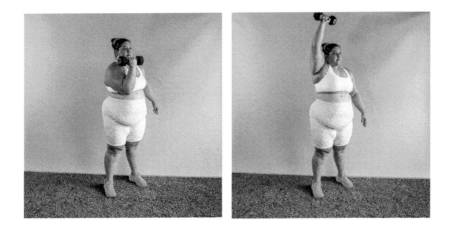

- Stand with your feet shoulder-width apart. Hold a dumbbell in each hand and rest them at shoulder height, with your elbows bent and palms facing your body.
- Slowly raise the dumbbells while rotating your wrists so that your palms are now facing forward (away from your body) until your arms are almost fully extended.
- Immediately begin lowering the dumbbells back down, rotating your wrists until your palms are now facing your body. Squeeze your chest at the bottom of each rep. Avoid bouncing the dumbbells together.

Modify Down
- Alternate arms and/or perform one arm at a time.

Modify Up
- Try a slightly heavier weight or add a resistance band.

Eccentric Dumbbell Hammer Curls

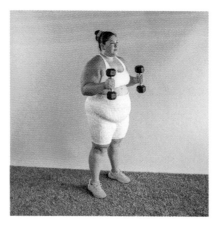

- Stand with your feet hip-width apart. Hold a dumbbell in each hand at your side with your palms facing your legs.
- Keeping your elbows tight at your sides, slowly bend your elbows by lifting your hands up toward your shoulders, keeping the dumbbells in a vertical position. Squeeze your biceps and pause for a moment at the top of each rep.
- Slowly straighten your elbows to lower the dumbbells back down to your sides as slowly as possible, taking a full four to five seconds per rep. Avoid swinging the dumbbells.

Modify Down
- Use lighter weights.
- Sit instead of standing.
- Use a light resistance band instead of dumbbells.

Modify Up
- Place a light resistance band under your feet and wrap around your dumbbells to create extra resistance as the weight is lifted.

Eccentric Dumbbell Lateral Raises

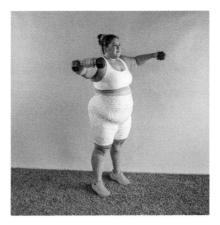

- Stand with your feet hip-width apart. Hold a dumbbell in each hand at your sides, with your palms facing your legs.
- With a slight bend in your elbows, slowly lift your arms out to the sides at shoulder level.
- Slowly lower your arms back to your sides as slowly as possible, taking a full four to five seconds per rep while keeping that same bend in your elbows. Avoid swinging the dumbbells.

Modify Down
- Use lighter weights.
- Sit on a bench instead of standing.
- Use a light resistance band instead of dumbbells.

Modify Up
- Place a light resistance band under your feet and wrap around your dumbbells to create extra resistance as the weight is lifted.

Back B

Five straight sets: Complete the first exercise for the full amount of sets before moving on to the next exercise. Rest as needed between sets and exercises, at least three to four minutes.

1. DB Reverse Flies *(5 sets, 10 reps)*
2. DB Straight Leg Dead Lifts *(5 sets, 10 reps)*
3. Bird Dog Crunches *(3 sets, 12 reps)*
4. DB Bent-Over Rows *(3 sets, 12 reps)*
5. Single DB Biceps Curls *(3 sets, 12 reps)*

Powerlift Option: Begin the workout with Barbell Dead Lifts, then continue through the rest of the workout (see page 172).

Dumbbell Reverse Flies

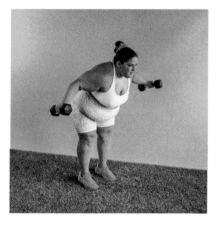

- Stand with your feet hip-width apart holding a dumbbell in each hand. Hinge forward at your hips until your torso is almost parallel with the ground. Allow the weights to hang down, palms facing each other.
- With a slight bend in your elbows, a flat back, and an engaged core, slowly lift the weights up and out to the sides until they're in line with your shoulders.
- Slowly lower them back down, keeping that same bend in your elbows. Momentum should be equal on the way up and on the way down. Avoid bouncing the dumbbells.

Modify Down
- Perform the move from a seated position.
- Use lighter weights or a light resistance band instead of dumbbells.

Modify Up
- Place a light resistance band under your feet and wrap around your dumbbells to create extra resistance as the weight is lifted.
- Place your feet in a lunge position while performing the exercise.

Dumbbell Straight Leg Dead Lifts

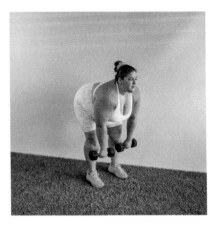

- Stand with your feet about shoulder-width apart. Hold a dumbbell in each hand in front of your waist, palms facing toward you.
- Keeping a slight bend in your knees, push your hips back and hinge forward until your torso is nearly parallel with the floor. Keep the dumbbells as close to your shins as possible throughout the entire move.
- Slowly move your hips forward to return back to the starting position.

Modify Down
- Use lighter weights.
- Use a light resistance band instead of dumbbells.

Modify Up
- Place a light resistance band under your feet and wrap around your dumbbells to create extra resistance as the weight is lifted.
- Try a single-leg dead lift by lifting one leg behind you as you hinge forward, balancing it parallel with the ground at the top of the move.

Bird Dog Crunches

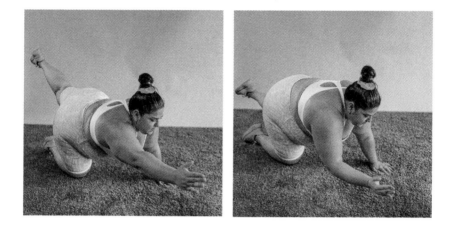

- Start with your hands and knees on the floor. Your knees should be under your hips with your wrists under your shoulders. Engage your core so your back is flat.
- Engaging your core to maintain a flat back, extend your right arm forward and left leg straight back, squeezing your left glute.
- Pull your right elbow and left knee in toward each other by squeezing your core. Finish the number of reps before reversing the movement on your other side.

Modify Down

- Use a higher incline such as a counter, bench, or sofa.

Modify Up

- Raise on your toes with your knees just a few inches above the ground throughout the entire exercise.

Dumbbell Bent-Over Rows

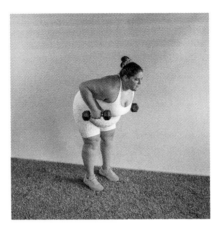

- Stand with your feet hip-width apart. Hold a dumbbell in each hand at your side with your palms facing your legs. Hinge forward at your hips, allowing your dumbbells to hang down in front of you.
- Engaging your core and squeezing your shoulder blades together, pull your elbows back and lift the dumbbells up toward the bottom of your chest. Keep your elbows close to your body.
- Pause and squeeze at the top before slowly lowering the dumbbells back to your starting position.

Modify Down
- Use lighter weights.
- Use a light resistance band instead of dumbbells.

Modify Up
- Place a light resistance band under your feet and wrap around your dumbbells to create extra resistance as the weight is lifted.

Single Dumbbell Biceps Curls

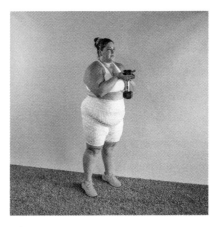

- Stand with your feet hip-width apart. Hold one dumbbell with both hands just under one end of the dumbbell (as if you're holding a plate).
- Keeping your elbows tight at your sides, slowly straighten your elbows by lowering your hands just enough to not let the top of your dumbbell tilt.
- Slowly bend your elbows by lifting your hands toward your chest. Squeeze your biceps and pause for a moment at the top of each rep.

Modify Down
- Use a lighter weight.

Modify Up
- Place a light resistance band under your feet and wrap around your dumbbell to create extra resistance as the weight is lifted.

Legs B

Three supersets: Complete the first and second exercises (1A and 1B) as one continuous set before resting and repeating for another set until all sets are complete. Then move on to the next superset (2A and 2B), followed by the final superset (3A and 3B). Rest as needed between sets and supersets, at least three to four minutes. Try not to pause for too long between superset A/B exercises.

1A. DB Goblet Squats *(4 sets, 8 reps)*

1B. DB Good Mornings *(4 sets, 8 reps)*

2A. DB Reverse Lunges *(3 sets, 10 reps)*

2B. Leg Raises *(3 sets, 10 reps)*

3A. Fire Hydrants *(2 sets, 12 reps/leg)*

3B. Butterfly Glute Bridges *(2 sets, 12 reps)*

Powerlift Option: Begin the workout with 10 to 15 slow and controlled Good Mornings (no dumbbell, hands at ears), followed by Barbell Back Squats instead of Goblet Squats (see page 167). Continue through the rest of the workout.

Dumbbell Goblet Squats

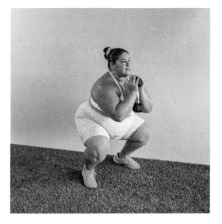

- Stand with your feet slightly wider than hip-width apart and your toes slightly turned outward. Hold a dumbbell vertically with both hands at chest level.
- Engaging your core while hinging at the hips first, bend your knees while lowering into a squat position where your thighs are either parallel or below parallel with the floor.
- Exhale and press heels into the ground to stand.

Modify Down
- Use lighter weights.
- Drop the dumbbells and do body-weight squats.
- Do a half squat, working your way down to a full squat as your strength and mobility begin to improve.
- Squat down into a chair.

Modify Up
- Use a resistance band around your thighs, just above your knees.

Dumbbell Good Mornings

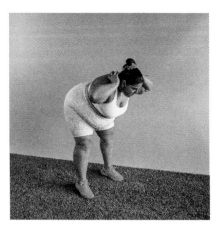

- Stand with your feet about shoulder-width apart. Hold one dumbbell horizontally behind your neck.
- Engaging your core and keeping your back flat, push your hips back and lower your torso until it is parallel to the floor.
- Pause, then return back to your starting position.

Modify Down

- Drop the dumbbell and use body weight only.

Modify Up

- Use a barbell or resistance band.

Dumbbell Reverse Lunges

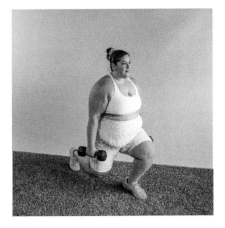

- Stand with your feet about shoulder-width apart. Hold a dumbbell in each hand at your sides with your palms facing your legs.
- Engaging your core and keeping your back straight, step backward with your right foot. Aim to land on the ball of your foot, with your heel off the ground. Bend both knees to about ninety degrees as you descend into a lunge.
- Push through the heel of your left foot to lift back to your starting position. Keep alternating between sides until your reps are complete for the set.

Modify Down
- Drop the dumbbells and use body weight only.
- Lower yourself only halfway, until your mobility and strength increase.

Modify Up
- Use a barbell instead of dumbbells.
- Try a reverse lunge holding a weight in just one hand.

Leg Raises

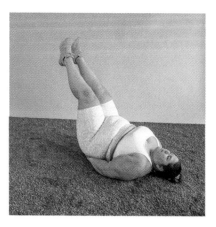

- Lie on your back with your legs straight and together, hands placed either under your butt or slightly out to the sides of your hips.
- Engaging your core, lift your legs all the way up toward the ceiling.
- Slowly lower your legs until they are just a few inches off the floor. Hold this for a moment before raising them again.

Modify Down

- Lift one leg at a time, keeping the other leg straight on the floor.

Modify Up

- Hold a dumbbell between your feet.

Fire Hydrants

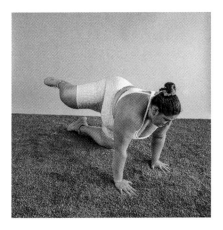

- Start with your hands and knees on the floor. Your knees should be under your hips with your wrists under your shoulders. Engage your core so your back is flat. Place a dumbbell behind your right knee.
- Keeping your right knee bent at ninety degrees, lift it out to the side as high as you can while engaging and lifting from your butt.
- Lower your leg back to the starting position. Repeat on the other leg.

Modify Down
- Drop the dumbbell and use body weight only.

Modify Up
- Add a resistance band around your thighs, just above your knees.

Butterfly Glute Bridges

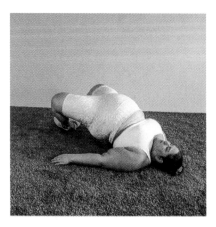

- Lie on your back with your feet together and knees pointed outward, creating a diamond shape with your legs.
- Engaging your core, drive your hips up in one controlled, yet explosive, movement.
- At the top squeeze your glutes before lowering your hips back to the starting position.

Modify Down

- Place your feet flat on the ground for a traditional hip thrust.

Modify Up

- Place a barbell, dumbbell, or sandbag across your lap, just above your hips.
- Add a resistance band around your thighs, just above your knees.

C WORKOUTS

Chest C

Three supersets: Complete the first and second exercise (1A and 1B) as one continuous set before resting and repeating for another set until all sets are complete. Then move on to the next superset (2A and 2B), followed by the final superset (3A and 3B). Rest as needed between sets and supersets, at least three to four minutes. Try not to pause for too long between superset A/B exercises.

1A. Eccentric DB Chest Press *(5 sets, 5 reps— slow on way down, pause, explode up)*

1B. Single DB Overhead Press *(5 sets, 10 reps)*

2A. DB Upright Rows *(4 sets, 10 reps)*

2B. DB Triceps Kickbacks *(4 sets, 10 reps)*

3A. Shrugs *(3 sets, 12 reps)*

3B. Up-Down Planks *(3 sets, 12 reps)*

Powerlift Option: Replace the Dumbbell Chest Press exercise with a Barbell Bench Press (see page 170).

Powerlift Option: Replace the Single Dumbbell Overhead Press with a Barbell Overhead Press with the barbell alone for 8 to 10 reps. Keep the superset as written, if possible. If a barbell is not available to immediately overhead press following bench press, use a single dumbbell as originally listed on the guide.

Eccentric Dumbbell Chest Press (see page 112)

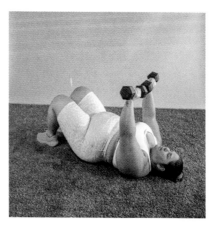

Choose slightly heavier weights. Lower the weights slowly (three to four counts) and explode on the way back up.

Dumbbell Overhead Press (see page 113)

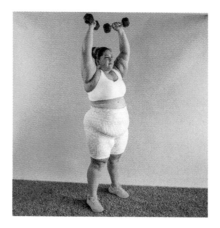

Dumbbell Upright Rows

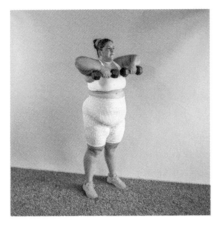

- Stand with your feet about shoulder-width apart. Hold a dumbbell in each hand in front of your waist, palms facing toward you.
- Slowly lift the dumbbells in front of you, keeping them close to your body until your elbows reach shoulder height.
- Slowly lower the dumbbells back to your starting position.

Modify Down
- Use lighter weights.
- Use a light resistance band instead of dumbbells.

Modify Up
- Place a light resistance band under your feet and wrap around your dumbbells to create extra resistance as the weight is lifted.

Dumbbell Triceps Kickbacks (see page 116)

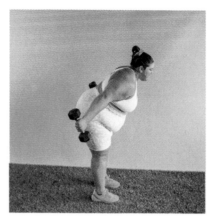

Shrugs

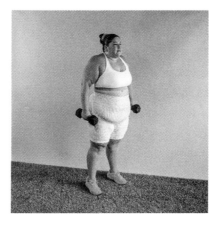

- Stand with your feet about shoulder-width apart. Hold a dumbbell in each hand at your sides with your palms facing your legs.
- Shrug your shoulders, keeping the weights completely still in your hands. Only your arms should be moving up and down through the shrug. (Think of pulling up and back at an angle rather than up and forward.)

Modify Down
- Use lighter weights.
- Use a light resistance band instead of dumbbells.

Modify Up
- Place a light resistance band under your feet and wrap around your dumbbells to create extra resistance as the weight is lifted.

Up-Down Planks

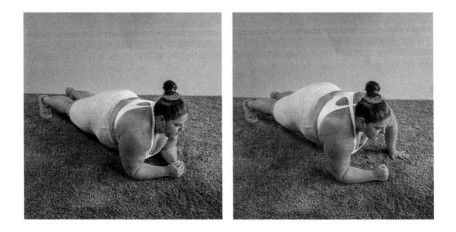

- In a high plank on the floor, place your hands shoulder-width apart, feet hip-width apart, and shoulders directly above your wrists.
- Engaging your core, lower yourself down into a forearm plank one arm at a time by lifting your right hand off the ground and placing your right forearm down on the ground. Repeat with your left arm.
- Raise yourself back up into a high-plank position by lifting your left forearm up off the ground and placing your left hand flat on the ground. Repeat with your right arm.

Modify Down
- Instead of a high plank on the ground, use a higher incline with a softer surface, such as a sofa or bed.

Modify Up
- Have a workout partner place a sandbag (or weighted bag) on your back for the duration of the exercise.

Back C

Five straight sets: Complete the first exercise for the full amount of sets before moving on to the next exercise. Rest as needed between sets and exercises, at least three to four minutes.

1. DB Bent-Over Rows *(5 drop sets, 15/12/10/8/6)*
2. Staggered Twisting Dead Lifts *(4 sets, 12 reps)*
3. Reverse Snow Angels *(4 sets, 12 reps)*
4. DB Biceps Curls *(4 sets, 12 reps)*
5. DB Sit-Up to Russian Twists *(4 sets, 12 reps)*

Powerlift Option: Begin the workout with Barbell Dead Lifts, then continue through the rest of the workout (see page 172).

Dumbbell Bent-Over Rows

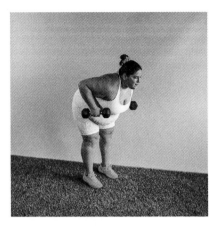

- Stand with your feet hip-width apart. Hold a dumbbell in each hand at your sides with your palms facing your legs. Hinge forward at your hips, allowing your dumbbells to hang down in front of you.
- Engaging your core and squeezing your shoulder blades together, pull your elbows back and lift the dumbbells toward the bottom of your chest. Keep your elbows close to your body.
- Pause and squeeze at the top before slowly lowering the dumbbells back down to your starting position.

Modify Down
- Use lighter weights.
- Use a light resistance band instead of dumbbells.

Modify Up
- Place a light resistance band under your feet and wrap around your dumbbells to create extra resistance as the weight is lifted.

Staggered Twisting Dead Lifts

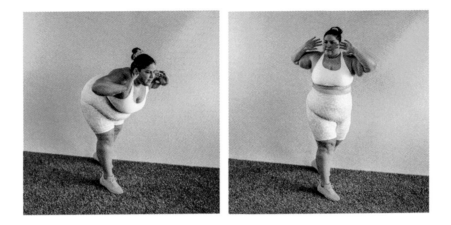

- Stand on your left leg, with your right leg placed behind you on your toes for balance and knees slightly bent. Place your hands by your ears, with your elbows open wide to the sides while squeezing your shoulder blades together.
- Engaging your core toward your spine and keeping your back straight, hinge forward from your hips until your torso is parallel (or as close to parallel as possible) to the floor.
- Press through your left heel and begin twisting your torso to the left as you back up to standing. Repeat for remaining reps before switching sides.

Modify Down
- Keep both feet together, shoulder-width apart, instead of staggering.

Modify Up
- Hold a light weight at your chest during the exercise.
- Add a resistance band around your thighs, just above your knees.

Reverse Snow Angels

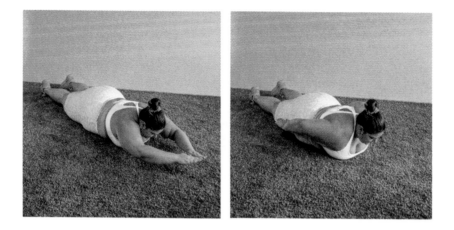

- Lie on your stomach with your arms extended above your head and palms facing down. Squeezing your glutes and lower back, raise your arms, chest, and legs slightly off the floor.
- Move your legs apart and your arms around down to your sides in a bow. Reverse the motion back to your starting position without letting any limbs touch the floor.
- Rest your limbs on the floor for a short moment before repeating the exercise.

Modify Down

- Perform one side at a time.

Modify Up

- Try not to let any limbs touch the ground between reps until the entire set is complete.

Dumbbell Biceps Curls

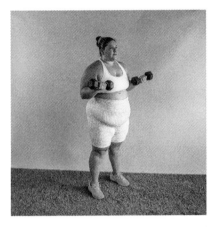

- Stand with your feet hip-width apart. Hold a dumbbell in each hand at your sides with your palms facing your legs.
- Keeping your elbows tight at your sides, slowly bend your elbows by lifting your hands up toward your shoulders and rotate the dumbbells so your palms face your chest. Squeeze your biceps and pause for a moment at the top of each rep.
- Slowly straighten your elbows to lower the dumbbells back down to your sides, rotating the weights so your palms are facing in toward your thighs. Avoid swinging the dumbbells.

Modify Down
- Use lighter weights.
- Sit on a bench instead of standing.
- Use a light resistance band instead of dumbbells.

Modify Up
- Place a light resistance band under your feet and wrap around your dumbbells to create extra resistance as the weight is lifted.

Dumbbell Sit-Up to Russian Twists

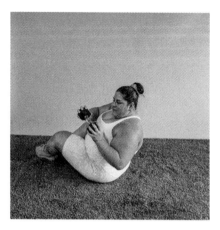

- Lie on your back with your knees bent and feet flat on the floor. Hold a single dumbbell horizontally at each end just above your chest.
- Engaging your core, curl your upper body all the way up toward your knees.
- Keeping the weight at chest level, continue engaging your core to twist from one side to the other before lowering back onto your back.

Modify Down
- Cross your feet for more stability.
- Drop the dumbbell and use body weight only, clasping your hands together.

Modify Up
- After sitting up, lift your feet off the ground during your twists.

Legs C

5 straight sets: Complete the first exercise for the full amount of sets before moving on to the next exercise. Rest as needed between sets and exercises, at least three to four minutes.

1. DB Tempo Squats *(5 sets, 5 reps—slow on the way down, pause)*
2. DB Donkey Kicks *(3 sets, 10 reps/leg)*
3. DB Forward Lunges *(3 sets, 10 reps/leg)*
4. DB Calf Raises *(3 sets, 20 reps)*
5. Scissors Kicks *(3 sets, 10 reps)*

Powerlift Option: Replace the Tempo Squats exercise with a Barbell Back Squat (see page 167).

Dumbbell Tempo Squats

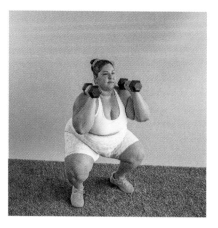

- Stand with your feet about shoulder-width apart and your toes slightly turned outward. Hold a dumbbell in each hand and rest them at shoulder height, with your elbows bent and palms facing each other.
- Engaging your core while hinging at the hips first, bend your knees while lowering your body into a squat position, where your thighs are either parallel or below parallel with the floor. As you're lowering, aim for a full four to five seconds to get you from standing into a squat position, before exploding on the way back up.
- Exhale and press heels into the ground to stand.

Modify Down
- Use lighter weights.
- Drop the dumbbells and do body-weight squats.
- Do a half squat, working your way down to a full squat as your strength and mobility begin to improve.
- Squat into a chair.

Modify Up

- Use heavier weights.
- Pause an extra two to three seconds at the bottom of your squat.

Dumbbell Donkey Kicks

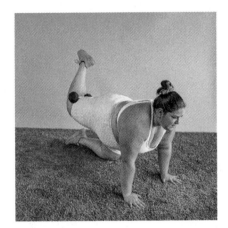

- Start with your hands and knees on the floor. Your knees should be under your hips with your wrists under your shoulders. Engage your core so your back is flat. Place a light dumbbell behind your right knee.
- Keeping your right knee bent at a ninety-degree angle, kick your right leg up into the air while engaging and lifting from your butt.
- Lower your leg back to the starting position. Repeat on the other leg.

Modify Down

- Drop the dumbbell and use your body weight only.

Modify Up

- Add a resistance band around your thighs, just above your knees.

Dumbbell Forward Lunges

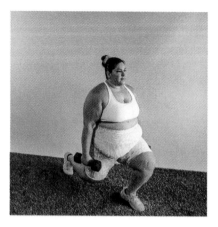

- Stand with your feet about shoulder-width apart. Hold a dumbbell in each hand at your sides with your palms facing your legs.
- Engaging your core and keeping your back straight, step forward with your right foot. Aim to land on the ball of your foot, with your heel off the ground. Bend both knees to about ninety degrees as you descend into a lunge.
- Push through the heel of your front foot to lift back to your starting position. Keep alternating between sides until your reps are complete for the set.

Modify Down
- Drop the dumbbells and use body weight only.
- Lower only halfway down, until your mobility and strength increase.

Modify Up
- Use a barbell instead of dumbbells.
- Try a forward lunge holding a weight in just one hand.

Dumbbell Calf Raises

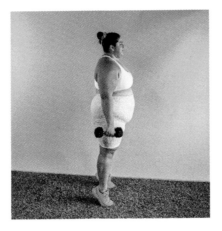

- Stand with your feet about hip-width apart. Hold a dumbbell in each hand at your sides with your palms facing your legs.
- Rise onto the balls of your feet as high as you can with control and squeezing your calves at the top.
- Pause, then lower back down slow and controlled.

Modify Down

- Drop the dumbbells and use body weight only.
- Hold on to a surface for support.
- Do the calf raises seated, with a pair of dumbbells lying on top of your knees.

Modify Up

- Do the calf raises a single leg at a time, holding one dumbbell with the opposite hand of the leg rising. Hold on to a surface for stability with your free hand. Perform equal reps on both sides.

Scissors Kicks

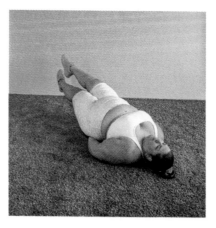

- Lie on your back with your legs straight and together, hands placed either under your butt or slightly out to the sides of your hips.
- Engaging your core and pressing your lower back into the floor, lift your legs a few inches above the floor, separating them slightly into a V shape.
- Keeping both legs straight, bring them closer together with your right foot crossing over your left. Then separate back into a V shape. This is 1 rep.

Modify Down

- Bend one leg and place it on the floor while the other leg performs the reps (in and out motions a few inches above the floor). Switch sides.

Modify Up

- Maintain a partial crunch (head and shoulders lifted off the floor with hands behind ears) throughout the entire set. Keep your neck neutral and avoid tucking your chin.

Self-Care Examples

- Foam rolling (see page 105)
- Yoga/meditation
- Mobility exercises
- Walk/jog
- Hot bath
- Massage
- Body image workshop
- Journaling

POWERLIFTING

Three lifts changed my life and introduced me to the world of powerlifting on an unforget-table evening in 2018. Squat, bench press, and dead lift are three beautiful compound movements (movements involving two or more body parts at once) that can seriously measure your strength. (And make you feel incredibly badass.) Powerlifting is a strength sport that consists of three single-rep attempts to lift as much weight as possible on squat, bench press, and dead lift.

First, let's smash some of the common misconceptions about powerlifting before we dive in. A lot of people automatically assume that powerlifting is all about getting as big and bulky as possible. Or that it's just a bunch of humans who were all born ridiculously strong and genetically built to push and pull some heavy-ass shit. (And if you don't think this applies to you, then there's no point in giving it a shot.) You may have even heard that it's superscary and dangerous. Well, nope, nope, and nope.

There are powerlifters of all shapes and sizes out there killing it, but the fitness industry rarely recognizes larger athletes outside of talking about their weight-loss journeys. So, I can understand why these misconceptions might be difficult to see beyond when you're deciding if powerlifting is worth exploring. I'm here to tell you, powerlifting is not just reserved for people with crazy strong genetics or people who want to compete. It's for all people who enjoy picking up heavy weights and want to feel strong in their bodies. And it's not dangerous if you focus on proper form and follow a well-designed program. Think about it. All other sports require you to focus on the task you're trying to accomplish, while remaining aware of your body and maneuvering it as safely as possible. Powerlifting is no different, and injuries are possible if proper form is ignored. But when done properly, powerlifting is one of the best ways for any athlete—from beginner to pro—to gain strength.

All right, so now that we know that powerlifting is for every body and everybody, let's chat about how to get started. If you're following my Twelve-Week Strength Training Guide, I have listed powerlifting options underneath each workout. There are also plenty of powerlifting programs available online. It can be a little overwhelming, especially if you're new to strength training and powerlifting. But here are a few important points to keep in mind and look for when deciding on what program might work best for you:

- **Number of reps:** Whether you're training to compete or to simply build your strength and do 1-rep max on all lifts, it's important to spend a good amount of your time powerlifting in the lower rep range (specifically, squat, bench press, and dead lifts). This is going to help build your strength toward a higher than 1-rep max.
- **Progressive overload:** Over time, you'll want to progressively increase the amount of weight you're lifting. You're trying to get your muscles to work harder as you get stronger.
- **Recovery/deload:** Rest is extremely important to incorporate into your training schedule. You want to avoid doing too much, too soon, when you first get started. One of the best recovery tools is scheduling deloads into your schedule, which is a scheduled period of time for you to take things a little easier and lighter than usual. This is going to help prevent injuries, plateaus, and just flat-out physical and mental exhaustion. Lots of information is online about what works best, but it's all about personal

preference. Maybe your body is asking for a full week off with light activities. Or maybe you plan for a deload week every eight to ten weeks of 30 to 50 percent of your 1-rep max for all lifts, while also cutting all of your sets in half that week. If you're a more experienced lifter, every six to eight weeks may work better for you. (Just remember, you're only deloading the amount of weight you're lifting, not the intensity of your lifts.) Another option is to keep the same amount of heavy weight you're lifting and decrease the number of sets and reps during a deload week.

Choosing the best powerlifting program for you depends on your specific goals, preferences, experience, and ability to recover. The program I follow (listed below) is based on what has worked well for me and my body after lots of experimenting, so if you choose to follow it, keep checking in with yourself about how your body is feeling. This program can easily be paired with the strength-training guide, but also live on its own. I additionally give a quick breakdown of each powerlift and all my best tips for how to use good form to give you the biggest strength gains!

Barbell Back Squat Prep and Form

Equipment Recommendations

- **Shoes**—hard soles with an elevated heel allowing you to push with your heel better
- **Wrist wraps**—eighteen to twenty-four inches long, wrapped a little above and below your wrist joint and tightened as much as comfortably possible
- **Belt**—10 to 13 mm and 4-inch-wide powerlifting belt worn just under your ribs, fastened about one notch looser than the tightest it will fit
- **Weight-lifting chalk**—placed on your upper back, allowing it to have a better grip under the bar
- **Knee sleeves**—warm your knee joints and provide enough pressure to feel secure

Form and Execution

- **Check your bar height on the rack.** The bar shouldn't be too high or too low. To check this, stand with your chest pressed up against the bar and lift your arms forward in front of you (think Frankenstein). The bar should be at the top of your breastbone, and about one to two inches below the height of the bar when it's on your back. You want to be able to unrack the bar without getting up on your tippy-toes, but also without having to squat down.

- **Position the bar on your back.** There are two different ways to position the bar, high-bar and low-bar. I tend to prefer low-bar on heavier lifts and high-bar on lighter lifts. There's no right or wrong way here—it's all based on what's comfortable for you.

  - In a *low-bar* position, the bar lies across your rear deltoid muscles. This works your hamstrings and glutes a little more and usually gives you more power (so you can lift more weight), but it's less comfortable. Since this position sits a little lower on your back, a little chalk dusted across your back can help the bar stick, and wrist wraps are a great way to help keep your wrists straight.

  - In a *high-bar* position, the bar lies across your traps (about two inches above low-bar) and works your quad muscles a little more. There is a bit less stress on your shoulders, while it allows you to get deeper into your squat. Just be careful in this position not to place the bar on your spine rather than your trap muscles. Get a feel for both and see which position is more comfortable for you.

- **Position your feet, grip, and unrack the bar.** Your hands should grip the bar as close to your shoulders as possible, where it's still comfortable. Your feet should be completely under the bar. Take a big, deep breath in, engage your core, and unrack the bar. Think about squeezing your glutes forward and using your quads, hips, hamstrings, and lower back to unrack the weight. Pause for a moment to let the weight settle before you begin stepping back.

- **Take three small, controlled steps back.** Start with one small step, allowing the weight to settle, followed by a second small step, allowing the weight to settle again. This second small step will plant your first foot down in your squatting position. Then take a third and final step back to plant your second foot to align with your other foot.

- **Adjust your stance and toe-point direction as needed.** I recommend a hip-width stance. If you're like me and have a larger midsection, it's important to adjust your stance a little wider to allow for a deeper squat, but not too wide, as that would compromise the rest of your form. Your toes should be pointed in a natural and comfortable position slightly outward. A fun way to check your natural toe position is to get into your squat stance and squeeze your glutes tight, then check where your toes landed.

- **Take a big, deep breath.** I mean *big*. Take in as much air as you can. I like to take a few quick seconds once I've gotten into my stance to take a few breaths leading up to my final, big inhale. All of these should get a little deeper and bigger each time. (This is my personal preference. You may benefit more from just a single big one.) The bigger and deeper your breath, the harder you can brace (push out your abdominal wall) and maintain a neutral spine throughout your lift (keeps you more upright with a straight back). This is where a belt comes in handy, allowing your core to have something to push up against as you brace and protect your lower back.

- **Drive your hips back to begin your squat.** Stand as if you're about to sit in a chair without bending forward, keeping your back as straight as you comfortably can.

- **Drive your knees out slightly as they bend.** Your knees should follow the same direction as and align with your toes without going farther than them throughout your squat.

- **After reaching your depth (parallel or below), drive your hips forward and squeeze your glutes through your lockout.** As you continue bracing your core (you still have that deep breath pushing out your abdominal wall), the first half of your lift back up should come naturally. On the second half, as soon as you start to struggle, try to focus more on driving your hips forward and seriously squeeze those glutes!

Barbell Bench Press Prep and Form

Equipment Recommendations

- **Shoes**—flat soles with a strong grip
- **Wrist wraps**—18 to 24 inches long, wrapped a little above and below your wrist joint and tightened as much as possible without causing you any pain or discomfort
- **Belt**—10 to 13 mm and 4-inch-wide powerlifting belt worn just under your ribs fastened about one notch looser than the tightest it will fit
- **Weight-lifting chalk**—placed on your upper back, allowing you to have a better grip on the bench

Form and Execution

- **Position your feet flat on the floor, as far back as you comfortably can.** I prefer to keep my feet placed a little farther back just below my butt to allow a small arch in my back. It's important to place your feet where you feel most comfortable while still having enough grip on the floor to create your base and avoid your feet moving around or kicking up. A flatter foot on the floor will provide a sturdier connection with the floor, so try to place your feet as far back as you can while still feeling sturdy. If you have shorter legs and can't quite reach the floor to feel sturdy enough, a thick bumper plate underneath each foot might just do the trick. (Or anything heavy and flat to raise the floor below your feet a few inches as needed.)
- **Position your back on the bench by aligning your forehead with the racked bar.** Your goal is to be able to reach the bar and unrack it comfortably (positioning too low on the bench will make this difficult), as

well as to not hit the rails as you press the bar up (positioning too high on the bench will make this inevitable). For me, lining up my forehead with the bar on the rack best positions my back on the bench; however, this will go a little differently for everyone, so play around until you find a position that works for you.

- **Arch your lower back slightly.** This tip tends to be controversial in the fitness community, but is only detrimental when done to the extreme. Creating a slight arch in your lower back is going to help keep your back tight and your spine neutral to protect it throughout your bench press. Sometimes powerlifters tend to arch their back drastically to create a shorter distance that the bar has to travel (to lift more weight for a bigger PR). This extreme type of arching isn't necessary for most, but a slight arch will help you engage your back and safely create the most power.

- **Grip the bar tightly, as far down into your hands as possible, with your thumb wrapped around the bar.** This will allow your wrists to remain straight throughout and provide the most power. Since we all have different bodies and arm lengths, each of us will grip at different widths. If your arms are longer, you'll probably grip the bar a little wider. Try not to exaggerate your grip in either direction. As a general guideline, aim to have your pinkie finger around the ring, or an inch or two more narrow.

- **Take a big, deep breath in and unrack the bar by squeezing your shoulder blades together and engaging your core.** Pull the bar off the rack in a slow and controlled manner. Imagine trying to squash a small grape between your shoulder blades while driving your shoulders into the bench. Your chest will naturally lift slightly, which will also help push the weight off the rack. Keep your shoulder blades squeezed and engaged throughout the entire bench press.

- **Take another big, deep breath in, engage your core, and begin to lower the weight toward your chest.** As you begin to lower the weight, imagine that you're trying to bend the bar into an upside-down *U* shape, allowing your elbows to naturally tuck in and lower the bar.

- **Touch the bar on your chest somewhere between your nipples and the top of your abs.** Since we all have different bodies, the exact positioning on this one will depend on your arm length. People with shorter arms and a wider grip will touch the bar a little higher up on their chest, closer to their nipples, while people with longer arms and a narrower grip will touch the bar a little lower on their chest, close to the top of their abs. Your main focus should be on keeping your forearms at a ninety-degree angle relative to the ground to avoid flaring your elbows. That will help you determine where you'll touch the bar on your body. Avoid bouncing the bar off your chest.

- **Squeeze your glutes, drive your feet into the ground, and exhale as you press the bar back up.** Doing this will give you more power to push the weight while keeping your body tight. As you push the weight, imagine that you're pushing it back toward the rack instead of straight up. As you lower the weight, keep your forearms perpendicular to the ground, so the bar lowers at a slight angle toward your chest. As you're pressing, you're simply reversing on the same track that you lowered in the opposite direction. Avoid rolling your shoulders forward as you lock out at the top.

Barbell Dead Lift Prep and Form

Equipment Recommendations

- **Shoes**—flat/thin soles with a strong grip
- **Long socks/pants**—to prevent you from scraping up your shins and thighs
- **Belt**—10 to 13 mm and 4-inch-wide powerlifting belt worn just under your ribs, fastened about one notch looser than the tightest it will fit
- **Weight-lifting chalk**—place on the palms of your hands allowing for a better grip on the bar and improving your overall grip strength (while also helping prevent the skin on your hands from tearing)
- **Choose your dead-lift setup either *conventional* or *sumo*.** Choose whichever you prefer, as both are equally beneficial. I tend to lean toward

a sumo dead-lift setup, but I still incorporate conventional dead lifts throughout my training. The biggest difference between the two is that they work a few different muscles.

Sumo Dead Lift Form

- **Position your feet at a wide-enough width so that your shins are perpendicular to the ground as you begin to pull.** An easy way to check this is to get in front of a mirror in your sumo starting position as if you're about to lift with your hands gripping the bar. You'll be able to clearly see just how wide you should place your feet by noting the angle of your shins. In your personal best sumo starting position, your shins will be at a ninety-degree angle to the ground. Move your feet around and see what kind of width works best for your body to achieve that angle.

- **Point your toes at a slight angle outward and position your hands straight down onto the bar.** This will allow the bar to lift as closely to your legs as possible without banging up your knees. I prefer using a mixed grip, where one hand is facing toward me (overhand) and one hand is facing away from me (underhand). Some people prefer an overhand grip only.

- **Take a big, deep breath in, engage your core and lats, and pull the slack out of the bar by driving your feet into the ground.** This simply means that you're tugging at the bar just enough to remove the slack (the weight is still on the ground) to help prevent your back from rounding and to keep the path of your bar straight. Imagine that you're spreading the floor apart rather than pushing the ground down. This is how you will begin your sumo dead lift.

Conventional Dead Lift Form

- **Position your feet about hip-width apart and your hands just outside your shins.** Or the width that would give you the most power if you were to try to jump as high as you can.

- **As you bend forward to grip the bar, keep your shins as perpendicular to the ground as possible while placing your hands just outside your shins.** Gripping too wide will force you to pull the bar an even farther distance, which is only going to make the dead lift more difficult. Focus on positioning your shoulders directly over the bar.

- **Take a big, deep breath in, engage your core and lats, and pull the slack out of the bar by driving your feet straight down into the ground.** This is similar to the sumo dead lift when pulling the slack out of the bar; however, this time imagine that you're bending the bar (also a similar thought process as in the bench press) and not only pulling the bar up, but also focusing on driving your feet straight into the ground (as opposed to sumo dead lifts, where you're pushing the ground apart). This is how you will begin your conventional dead lift.

Sumo and Conventional Dead Lift Execution

- **Squeeze your glutes and drive your hips forward as the bar begins to lift up off the ground, while keeping the bar as close to your shins as possible.** This will feel different depending on if you're doing a sumo or conventional dead lift. Sumo will most likely lift off the ground a bit slower, while conventional will most likely lift up a bit faster when using proper form. As with squat and bench press, a belt will give you something to press your abdominal wall against when you engage your core and aim to keep your back upright during the dead lift.

- **Lock out your lower back by continuing to squeeze your glutes.** Avoid overextending your lower body and aim to stand as straight as possible during your lockout, while also not allowing your knees to lock out too soon. They should lock out at about the same time the rest of your lower body does.

- **Lower the bar in a controlled manner, without dropping it, and drive your hips back.** Focus on lowering the bar down that same straight bar path that you lifted it on.

- **Allow the weight and the bar to settle between reps.** Avoid bouncing the bar on the ground in between reps. The best thing you can do to get the most out of every rep is allow the weight to settle on the ground (keeping your grip) and lifting the dead weight on your next rep. If you're up for even more of a challenge, let go of your grip and stand back up straight for two to three seconds before completely resetting for your next rep.

Barbell Overhead Press Prep and Form

- **Check your bar height on the rack.** The bar shouldn't be too high or too low. To check this, stand with your chest pressed up against the bar. It should be pressed up against the top of your clavicle.
- **Position your feet and your grip.** Your hands should grip the bar tightly, just a little wider than shoulder-width apart, and as far down into your hands as possible, with your thumb wrapped around the bar and elbows angled slightly down. Your feet should be completely under the bar about shoulder-width apart.
- **Take a big, deep breath in, engage your core, and unrack the bar.** Think about squeezing your glutes forward and using your quads, hips, hamstrings, and lower back to unrack the weight. Pause for a moment to let the weight settle before you begin stepping back. Take a few small and controlled steps back to stand in your starting position, with the bar on top of your clavicle and your hips stacked under the bar.
- **Take another big, deep breath in and tuck your chin up and back as you begin to press the bar up over your head while maintaining a straight line.** Think of it like giving yourself a double chin to allow your face to be out of the way for you to push the bar up in a straight line.
- **Once the bar passes your face and you're locked out above your head, focus on your vertical alignment, which should be the bar, your shoulders, and the front of your hips.** Avoid sticking out your butt or pushing the bar up and away from your body as you press. Your head

should be tucked in between your arms (meaning your ears will most likely be visible in front of your arms when you're locked out). This will engage the muscles in your upper back, which is going to help you lift more weight safely and gain overall strength in your shoulders.

- **As you lower the weight, tuck your chin up and back in the same position as before.** This will also allow the bar to descend on that same straight-line path without hitting you in the head. Allow the weight to settle before continuing on to the next rep or stepping forward to place the bar back on the rack.

Choose a starting weight for bench press, overhead press, and squat with which you can do three sets of 5 reps fairly easily. Choose a starting weight for dead lift where you can do one set of 5 reps fairly easily. It might take a little experimenting if you're new to powerlifting. If you're not a beginner and you know you're currently at 1-rep max on all of your lifts, your working weight to begin the program should be around 75 percent of your 1-rep max. Your working weight will always be the final group of sets you will perform on squats, bench press, and dead lifts. (I'm adding overhead press as well since it's helped me tremendously with my shoulder strength!) Each session will begin with the barbell alone for two warm-up sets on all lifts except dead lifts.

To calculate your **squat** sets, start with 40 percent of your working weight. Follow that up with 60 percent and then 80 percent for the rest of the warm-up sets. Each leg day (or squat day if you aren't following the strength-training guide in this book), you will increase your working weight by five pounds, which will give you all new weights for your warm-up sets each session. Here's a quick breakdown:

1. Warm-up with barbell: *2 sets, 5 reps*
2. Warm-up at 40 percent: *1 set, 5 reps*
3. Warm-up at 60 percent: *1 set, 3 reps*
4. Warm-up at 80 percent: *1 set, 2 reps*
5. Working weight: *3 sets, 5 reps*

Example Squat Session 1, 135 pounds working weight

1. Barbell: *2 sets, 5 reps*
2. 40 percent, 55 pounds: *1 set, 5 reps (grab an extra set of the barbell alone if your 40 percent is currently below 45 pounds)*
3. 60 percent, 80 pounds: *1 set, 3 reps*
4. 80 percent, 105 pounds: *1 set, 2 reps*
5. Working weight, 135 pounds: *3 sets, 5 reps*

Example Squat Session 2, 140* pounds working weight
*Increased working weight by 5 pounds

1. Barbell: *2 sets, 5 reps*
2. 40 percent, 55 pounds: *1 set, 5 reps (grab an extra set of the barbell alone if your 40 percent is currently below 45 pounds)*
3. 60 percent, 80 pounds: *1 set, 3 reps*
4. 80 percent, 110 pounds: *1 set, 2 reps*
5. Working weight, 140 pounds: *3 sets, 5 reps*

To calculate your **bench press** sets, start with 50 percent of your working weight. Follow that up with 70 percent and then 90 percent for the rest of the warm-up sets. Each chest day, you will increase your working weight by five pounds, which will give you all new weights for your warm-up sets each session. Here it is broken out:

1. Warm-up with barbell: *2 sets, 5 reps*
2. Warm-up at 50 percent: *1 set, 5 reps*
3. Warm-up at 70 percent: *1 set, 3 reps*
4. Warm-up at 90 percent: *1 set, 2 reps*
5. Working weight: *3 sets, 5 reps*

Example Bench Press Session 1, 80 pounds working weight

1. Barbell: *2 sets, 5 reps*
2. 50 percent, 40 pounds: *1 set, 5 reps (grab an extra set of the barbell alone if your 50 percent is currently below 45 pounds)*

3. 70 percent, 55 pounds: *1 set, 3 reps*
4. 90 percent, 70 pounds: *1 set, 2 reps*
5. Working weight, 80 pounds: *3 sets, 5 reps*

Example Bench Press Session 2, 85* pounds working weight
*Increased working weight by 5 pounds

1. Barbell: *2 sets, 5 reps*
2. 50 percent, 40 pounds: *1 set, 5 reps (grab an extra set of the barbell alone if your 50 percent is currently below 45 pounds)*
3. 70 percent, 60 pounds: *1 set, 3 reps*
4. 90 percent, 75 pounds: *1 set, 2 reps*
5. Working weight, 85 pounds: *3 sets, 5 reps*

To calculate your **dead lift** sets, take 40 percent of your working weight. Follow that up with 60 percent and then 85 percent for the rest of the warm-up sets. Each back day (or dead-lift day if you aren't following the strength-training guide in this book), you will increase your working weight by ten pounds, which will give you all new weights for your warm-up sets each session. Here it is broken down:

1. Warm-up at 40 percent: *2 sets, 5 reps*
2. Warm-up at 60 percent: *1 set, 3 reps*
3. Warm-up at 85 percent: *1 set, 2 reps*
4. Working weight: *3 sets, 5 reps*

Example Dead-Lift Session 1, 100 pounds working weight

1. 40 percent, 40 pounds: *2 sets, 5 reps (two sets of the barbell alone if your 40 percent is currently below 45 pounds)*
2. 60 percent, 60 pounds: *1 set, 3 reps*
3. 85 percent, 85 pounds: *1 set, 2 reps*
4. Working weight, 100 pounds: *3 sets, 5 reps*

Example Dead-Lift Session 2, 110* pounds working weight

Increased working weight by 10 pounds

1. 40 percent, 45 pounds: *2 sets, 5 reps (two sets of the barbell alone if your 40 percent is currently below 45 pounds)*
2. 60 percent, 65 pounds: *1 set, 3 reps*
3. 85 percent, 90 pounds: *1 set, 2 reps*
4. Working weight, 110 pounds: *3 sets, 5 reps*

This would continue for the duration of the twelve weeks: increasing your working weight by five pounds at every chest session. If you don't have the right weight increments to add to the bar based on the percentage, either round up or down depending on how you're feeling that day. I also usually attempt a true 1-rep max every other week, but how you proceed is totally up to you and your comfort level. Just make sure you have someone who can spot you before deciding to go for an attempt. Once I complete all of my sets, depending on how I feel, I will add another set and attempt a single rep that is close or equal to my current 1-rep max. If I don't think I have enough left in the tank to complete my working weight sets, I'll skip the single. Once the twelve weeks are complete and you're preparing for another round, you can switch things up every now and then by adding resistance bands, trying midway pauses, or even replacing your working-weight sets with sets of heavy singles. No matter what, I definitely recommend sticking to the program for at least the first twelve weeks, especially if you're new to powerlifting. It will more than likely give you the biggest opportunity for lots of strength gains! Don't worry if there's a week you don't hit all your sets and reps with the five-pound increase in weight. Try the same working weight again the next session and don't move up in weight until you've completed the sets without reaching failure. Everyone is different (remember to allow yourself to rest and recover!), so if you go a couple of sessions before increasing your weight, it's okay! The more you focus on good form, recovering, and having fun, the more you'll start to feel your strength building! You got this!

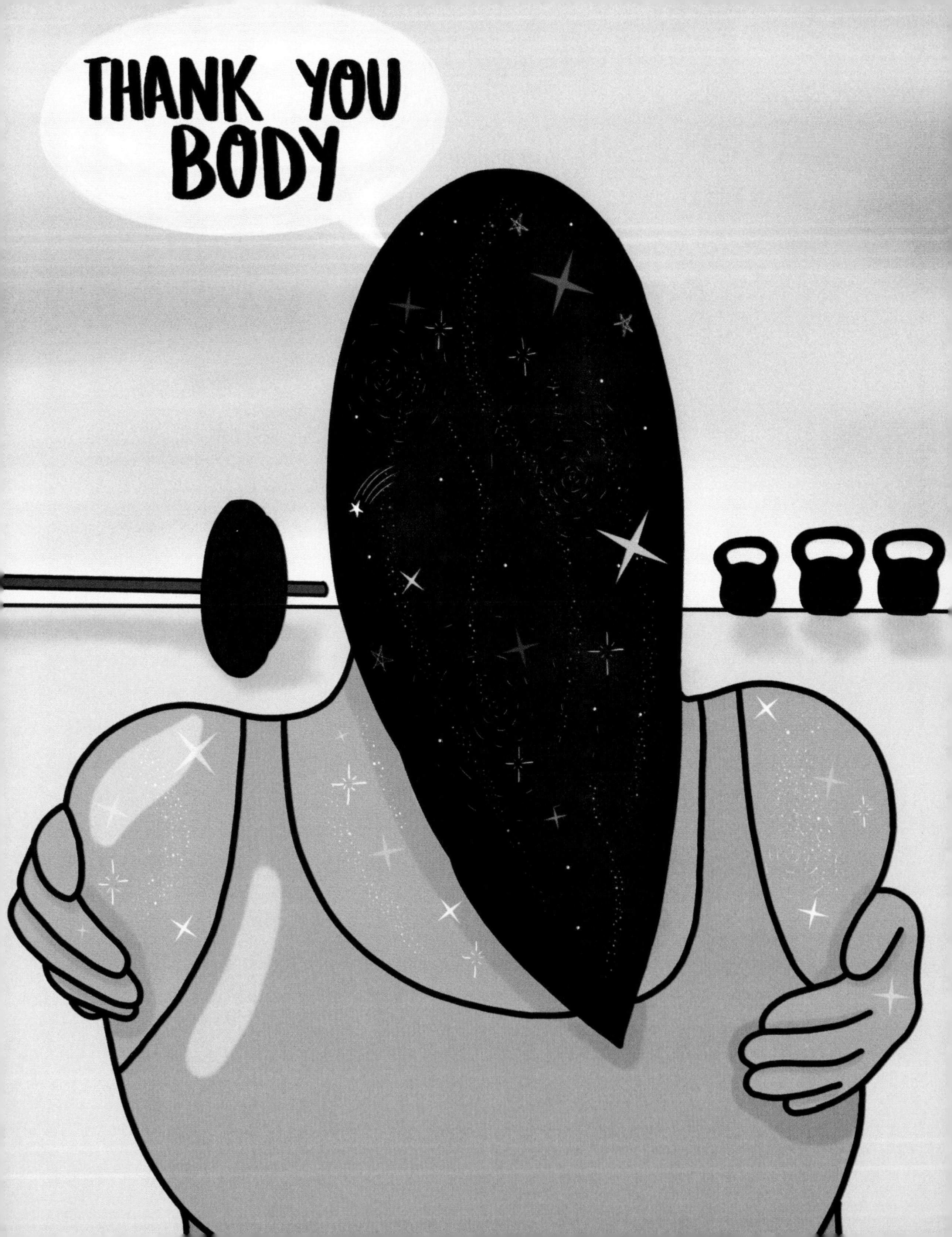
THANK YOU BODY

Part 6

The Part Where We Remember Our Worth

The roll above the bend of my elbow disappeared for the year between my weight loss and when I got pregnant. Those were my skinniest days, which were also my darkest. I still don't quite understand why I cared about this roll or why it mattered to me. I don't know why it caused me to always pull at my shirtsleeves to make sure it was covered up. Or why sleeveless tops made me feel naked, as if I were always worried about the world finding out that I was fat and had rolls on my arms. Or rolls on my back. Or rolls on my upper thighs. I used shirt tugging and arm crossing and baggy clothes as my crutch. When the roll above the bend of my elbow began to shrink with weight loss, it left a line. It left proof. The line took the place of the roll, continuing to fill my heart with hate and disgust. It was an intense and constant embarrassment-filled ache. As my belly grew life, the line transitioned back into a roll.

I Have Rolls

I have rolls.

I have anxiety.

I get hopeful.

I get scared.

I have feelings that run deep and it's taken me
years to finally share.

I've had fears around love and allowing self-love
to begin.

I've questioned my self-worth when I feel the
depression kick in.

I'm a little bit different.

And yet so much the same.

I haven't always understood it.

But the truth in it all remains.

I have rolls.

I have anxiety.

I get hopeful.

I get scared.

And yet I'm still beautifully, interestingly, and
    most definitely rare.

As I've mentioned, I'd like to think I had a magical aha moment that extended beyond the birth of my daughter. But I didn't. The closest I came to that moment was when I grabbed that pair of scissors and cut off the sleeves of several tees that became my workout tanks. But even in that moment, I wasn't ready. Yet I cut the sleeves off anyway, scissors shaking in my hands. I'd also like to think those uncomfortable, not-ready moments were more about growth than magic. Sometimes I still glance down and get a few nervous butterflies as I see the rolls on my arms, revealing themselves to everyone around me as I'm in between sets. But then my eyes shift back to my workout because I see the shit ton of weight that these rolls can lift. And I can't help but kind of just be, like, *You go, roll. You fucking go.*

So, sure. I have rolls on my body. I also have happiness and memories and life; that is special and worth being seen. The more of us that allow ourselves to be seen, the more the world around us is exposed to just how fascinating and incredible our differences make us. In our squishiness. And in our colorfulness. And in our unapologetic realness.

I'm not looking to achieve a measurable amount of acceptance from anyone or anything. Some days I struggle so fucking much that I reach for my phone, look down, and snap a photo. Because I know it might just mean something to me on another day. So I weep. I have a moment when I fully allow myself to break. This is instead of saying the words "This is beautiful" on repeat; instead of pretending that I have this all figured out and I'm setting some sort of perfect example; instead of holding it all in. Because in the midst of the madness and fear and sometimes even rage, I fight to keep going. Because while the pre-baby me worked hard for a smaller pant size, the postbaby me worked even harder to appreciate the pant size she's currently in. And because I am allowed to weep and break during the moments that swallow me whole. Because I am human. I have a belly full of stretch marks, for whatever reasons. I also have them all over my boobs, and across my hips, and on my thighs, and arms, and in all kinds of places on my body where they appeared before I can even remember.

Sometimes when we lean into our softness, even when things feel hard, we find the part of ourselves that holds the greatest power. It's the moments in which we feel vulnerable that we get an opportunity to demonstrate strength, by simply being, while allowing those around us to simply be, too. Uncomfortable conversations that are new, especially when they are conversations that you have with yourself, can feel scary. We can either choose to embrace them with curiosity or dismiss them through our own ignorance. But when we neglect these new ideas, we miss a beautiful realization: that it is possible to discover strength in softness. But it can't be done without the discomfort of learning and unlearning and truly leaning into those hard as hell moments of opportunity and growth.

So, sure, a lot of us have stretchy and wrinkly and dimply odd-shaped bits. A lot of us are soft. But, you know what? That's exactly the kind of shit that makes you so damn strong.

THE THANK-YOUS

I used to weigh my body every morning. I would always make sure to go to the bathroom first. There would be this giant rush of anxiety as the scale blinked while I stared down in anticipation. This moment would decide how I approached my day. Would I be positive and embrace the day happily because the number was a whole 0.1 ounces lower than yesterday morning? Or would I angrily start brushing my teeth and threaten myself with only eating salad for the day because the number was a whole 0.1 ounces higher than yesterday? This was how I lived each and every day for years, and it was slowly destroying every part of me. But then there she was, my Maci Ann. For the first time, I felt an ounce of thankfulness for my body. I had that tiny taste of what it might feel like to live a life of liberation in my body.

After she was born, I stood for a moment in the hospital bathroom just before I took my first postpartum shower. I stood in my robe as I stared into the mirror. I had avoided mirrors for years, even throughout most of my pregnancy. Locking eyes with myself, I tugged the string and the robe separated a few inches. I froze for a few seconds before I let the robe fall to the floor. And there I was. I saw me for what felt like the very first time, but after another few seconds, I closed my eyes and began to sob. I turned around and walked toward the shower. I knew that I felt something deep, but I didn't realize it was the seed of something much bigger. It was the start of an inner revolution. The very first thank you.

The Softness
It Just Is, I Just Am

I would say that it's because of pregnancy and postpartum, but it's not.

I would say that it's because of my age, but it's not.

I would say that it's because of the two years I spent losing a lot of weight, but it's not.

I would say that it's because I do a lot of chest workouts, but it's not.

I would say that it's because of the way I fuel my body, but it's not.

I would say that it's because of whatever lie I've been made to believe, but it's not.

It's just because that's how they are. And how my body is.

Without need for reasons. Or defenses.

Without internal justifications used to create internal gratifications before eventually forcing myself into the need for external modifications.

Could there be reasons they've always been the way they are?

These sagging boobs and these stretch-marked hips.

Maybe? Maybe not? Who literally cares?

It just is.

I just am.

And I'm no longer afraid of being who I'm currently meant to be.

Normalcy mixed with a one-of-a-kind me.

When you grow up in a fat body, chances are you're made fun of for every single thing you do. The most basic shit like how you breathe or how you walk or what you eat. People make fun of you when you dance or when you sit, and even if you run a marathon or lift heavy weights. They make fun of you when you find love or land the dream job. In a fat body, you are never allowed to have one accomplishment celebrated openly (making your body smaller) without it somehow becoming a joke. So, you eventually stop dancing. You stop laughing and smiling for pictures (if you even find the courage to be in them). You stay home. You cover up. You hide. You stop pursuing your dreams and start pursuing weight loss. You live with this overwhelming deep-rooted embarrassment.

It's ridiculous and dehumanizing. It's paralyzing because that mind-set invades every facet of your life. But then a moment presents itself to you in a way you may not recognize at first. You won't be looking for it, but the whole time it's been looking for you in quick glances as you walk by mirrors; in a belly laugh when you forget for a moment how laughing makes your belly shake; in every tiny moment you were completely unaware of the way your body began producing sweat knowing full well you needed a cooldown in the middle of that scorching summer heat; in your breath as you whisper the words, "I love you," for the very first time; in the way you begin to not think twice about the volume of your breath. Because in those small moments, magic happens. You remember what it's like to dance, to laugh, to run and jump, to lift, smile, and live. So finally, you exhale. You begin to move your body in ways that make you happy. You are no longer convinced that your body has no worth. You are no longer convinced that focusing on strength just isn't for someone like you. You are no longer someone who thinks you could never be strong. You are no longer someone who thinks you should just focus on losing weight. You are someone who never stops doing the things you love. Because you always knew deep down that none of that shit has ever been true.

SO, SHOW UP

Show up even when you're met with criticism. Even when people want more from you. Even when finding motivation outside of societal demands seems impossible. Even when your hair is messy. Even when you aren't the strongest or fastest human on earth. Even when you're not wearing makeup. Even when your outfit doesn't match. Even when you're covered in body hair. Even when it's overwhelming to face your fears. Even when you don't feel ready. Even when you don't believe it's possible. Even when the comments you overhear or see about you still seem to never stop sounding like nails on a chalkboard in familiar yet always unexpected ways. Show up anyway.

Show up in moments when people's words evolve into the words you begin gathering as your own and interrupt them loudly. Show up in moments you forget that *you* are what's important here. Be daring. Stand taller. Be scared. Own it. Take the photo. Wear the swimsuit. Eat the pizza. (If you like pizza.) Or the salad with guacamole. (If you like salad and guacamole.) Show up for the girls' night out. Read the book. Ask for help. Jump in the pool. Call people back (or text them because they're millennials). Dance in your underwear. Look in the mirror. Give yourself the chance to do the things you love and love the things you are. Whatever you do in these moments that swallow you whole and create thunder in your memory, I hope you choose you. Because, honey, you were made from magic. Whatever you do, don't allow yourself to be one of the ones choosing to cover up all of that magic, too.

Stand tall and then stand taller. Dream loud and then dream louder. Show up loud and then show up louder. When they call you thunder, allow your storm to keep growing. Then let it fucking roar. It will feel scary at first. Do it anyway.

Dear Body,

I'm sorry I didn't trust you.

I'm sorry I ignored you when all you were trying to do was survive.

(And, gosh, I'm so sorry that I would punish you for that.)

I'm sorry I felt so disgusted by you.

I'm sorry I said terrible things about you.

I'm sorry that out of shame I covered you in old, baggy clothes that I hated.

I'm sorry I told you that swimsuits weren't for you.

I'm sorry I bought that weird thing that promised to scrub away your dimples and only caused you pain.

I'm sorry I ingested every toxic chemical in hopes you would morph into anything else but you.

I'm sorry I allowed myself to be convinced that you were wrong.

I'm sorry that I have to constantly defend you when you are so worthy of respect.

I'm sorry we have to experience life in a society that chooses to not always see what I see and openly vocalizes the reasons why you should change.

Because I see the beauty in your humanity.

I see a body that breathes life and love.

A body that is doing everything possible to keep me alive.

To keep me experiencing.

To keep me doing the things that I love.

I'm sorry I didn't see that and appreciate it until now.

(I'm also sorry that I still have days when it's hard for me and I find myself feeling triggered by an old narrative. But I promise that I'm always trying.)

I'm just so incredibly sorry for it all.

And wanted to say thank you.

You never quit on me.

Even after I repeatedly quit on you.

So even though there's a lot for me to feel sorry about, there's a lot more for me to feel thankful for.

Thank you, body—for literally everything

Additional Resources

HEALTH / INTUITIVE EATING / ANTI-DIET / EATING DISORDER RECOVERY

Books

Bacon, Lindo. *Health at Every Size: The Surprising Truth about Your Weight*. Dallas, TX: BenBella Books, 2010.

Dooner, Caroline. *The F*ck It Diet: Eating Should Be Easy*. New York: HarperCollins, 2019.

Harrison, Christy. *Anti-Diet: Reclaim Your Time, Money, Well-Being, and Happiness through Intuitive Eating*. New York: Little, Brown Spark, 2019.

Saunt, Rosie, and Helen West. *Is Butter a Carb?: Unpicking Fact from Fiction in the World of Nutrition*. London: Piatkus, 2019.

Thomas, Laura. *Just Eat It: How Intuitive Eating Can Help You Get Your Shit Together around Food*. London: Bluebird, 2019.

Tribole, Evelyn. *Intuitive Eating: A Revolutionary Anti-Diet Approach*. 4th ed. New York: St. Martin's Essentials, 2020. (@evelyntribole)

Turner, Pixie. *The Insta-Food Diet: How Social Media Has Shaped the Way We Eat*. London: Anima, 2020.

Podcasts

Ackerman, Kirsten. "Intuitive Bites." https://podcasts.apple.com/us/podcast/intuitive-bites-podcast/id1383888050?mt=2.

"The Anti-Diet Plan." https://www.theantidietplan.com/.

Dooner, Caroline. "The F*ck It Diet." https://podcasts.apple.com/us/podcast/the-f-ck-it-diet-with-caroline-dooner/id1084208738.

"The Eating Disorder Center." Eating Disorder Center. https://www.theeatingdisordercenter.com/.

Goodman, Rachel. "More Than What You Eat." https://podcasts.apple.com/us/podcast/more-than-what-you-eat/id1464580727.

Harrison, Christy. "Food Psych." https://podcasts.apple.com/us/podcast/food-psych-intuitive-eating/id700512884.

Jones, Jessica, and Wendy Lopez. "Food Heaven: The Podcast." *Dear Media*. https://podcasts.apple.com/us/podcast/food-heaven-podcast/id1041814489.

National Eating Disorders Association. https://www.nationaleatingdisorders.org/.

"The Original Intuitive Eating Pros." Intuitive Eating. http://www.intuitiveeating.org/.

Thomas, Laura. "Don't Salt My Game." https://podcasts.apple.com/us/podcast/dont-salt
-my-game-with-laura-thomas-phd/id1111787243.

Websites

- www.neda.com (@neda), National Eating Disorders Association
- www.intuitiveeating.org
- www.theantidietplan.com (@theantidietplan)
- www.theeatingdisordercenter.com (@theeatingdisordercenter)

Instagram Must-Follows

- @jennifer_rollin
- @theshirarose
- @thenutritiontea
- @your.latina.nutritionist
- @kristamurias
- @fitfatandallthat
- @dietitiananna
- @drjoshuawolrich
- @workweeklunch
- @nourishandeat
- @antidietriotclub
- @thefuckitdiet
- @laurathomasphd
- @rooted_project
- @pixienutrition
- @lucymountain
- @chr1styharrison
- @theintuitive_rd
- @dietitian.rachelgoodman
- @foodheaven

BODY IMAGE / SELF-CONFIDENCE / FAT ACTIVISM / MENTAL HEALTH

Books

Baker, Jes. *Things No One Will Tell Fat Girls: A Handbook of Unapologetic Living.* Berkeley, CA: Seal Press, 2015.

Crabbe, Megan Jayne. *Body Positive Power: Because Life Is Already Happening and You Don't Need to Lose Weight to Live It.* Berkeley, CA: Seal Press, 2018.

Crenshaw, Katie, and Ady Meschke. *Her Body Can.* Houston, TX: East 26th Publishing, 2020.

Elman, Michelle. *Am I Ugly?* London: Head of Zeus, 2018.

Hagen, Sofie. *Happy Fat: Taking Up Space in a World That Wants to Shrink You.* New York: HarperCollins, 2020.

Strings, Sabrina. *Fearing the Black Body: The Racial Origins of Fat Phobia.* New York: NYU Press, 2019.

Taylor, Sonya Renee. *The Body Is Not an Apology: The Power of Radical Self-Love.* Oakland, CA: Berrett-Koehler, 2018.

Yeboah, Stephanie. *Fattily Ever After: The Fat, Black Girls´ Guide to Living Life Unapologetically.* London: Hardie Grant Books, 2020.

Podcasts

Brenna, Kenzie. "Conversations with Kenzie." https://podcasts.apple.com/us/podcast /conversations-with-kenzie/id1509586423.

Brown, Brené. "Unlocking Us." *Brené Brown and Cadence 13*. https://podcasts.apple .com/us/podcast/unlocking-us-with-bren%C3%A9-brown/id1494350511.

Carter-Kahn, Sophie. "She's All Fat." https://podcasts.apple.com/us/podcast/shes-all -fat-a-fat-positive-podcast/id1275942047.

Gaudreau, Steph. "Listen to Your Body." https://podcasts.apple.com/us/podcast /listen-to-your-body-podcast/id999471212.

Gordon, Aubrey, and Michael Hobbes. "Maintenance Phase." https://podcasts.apple .com/us/podcast/maintenance-phase/id1535408667

Jamil, Jameela. "I Weigh." *Earwolf*. https://podcasts.apple.com/us/podcast/i-weigh -with-jameela-jamil/id1498855031.

Scritchfield, Rebecca. "Body Kindness." https://podcasts.apple.com/us/podcast/body -kindness/id1073275062.

Treloar, Erin. "Raw Beauty Talks." https://podcasts.apple.com/us/podcast/raw-beauty -talks/id1454866000.

Instagram Must-Follows

- @effyourbeautystandards
- @fatgirlflow
- @arti.speaks
- @arielleestoria
- @bodyimage_therapist
- @tiffanyima
- @yrfatfriend
- @wheelchair_rapunzel
- @iamdaniadriana
- @beauty_redefined
- @roseybeeme
- @meghantonjes
- @therapyforblackgirls
- @fatpositivetherapy
- @decolonizingtherapy
- @therapyforwomen
- @sonyareneetaylor
- @bodyposipanda
- @sofiehagendk
- @themilitantbaker
- @stephanieyeboah
- @scarrednotscared
- @i_weigh
- @shesallfatpod
- @rawbeautytalks
- @kenziebrenna
- @pinkmantaray
- @torii.block

MOTHERHOOD / PLUS-SIZE PREGNANCY AND POSTPARTUM / FERTILITY

Books

Huntpalmer, Bryn. *The First-Time Mom's Pregnancy Handbook: A Week-by-Week Guide from Conception through Baby's First 3 Months*. Emeryville, CA: Rockridge Press, 2019.

Koziol, Jill, and Liz Tenety. *This Is Motherhood: A Motherly Collection of Reflections + Practices*. Louisville, CO: Sounds True, 2019.

McLellan, Jen. *My Plus Size Pregnancy Guide: Stop Googling and Start Feeling Empowered*. Scotts Valley, CA: CreateSpace, 2016.

Salmon, Nicola. *Fat and Fertile: How to Get Pregnant in a Bigger Body*. Self-published, 2019.

Podcasts

Belknap, Catherine, and Natalie Telfer. "#MOMTRUTHS with Cat & Nat." https://podcasts.apple.com/us/podcast/momtruths-with-cat-nat/id1439920596.

Erica and Milah. "Good Moms Bad Choices." https://podcasts.apple.com/us/podcast/good-moms-bad-choices/id1356670998.

Huntpalmer, Bryn. "The Birth Hour—a Birth Story Podcast." https://podcasts.apple.com /us/podcast/the-birth-hour-a-birth-story-podcast/id1041801905.

Masony, Meredith, and Tiffany Jenkins. "Take It or Leave It." https://podcasts.apple .com/us/podcast/take-it-or-leave-it/id1434126027.

McLellan, Jen. "Plus Mommy Podcast." https://podcasts.apple.com/us/podcast/plus -mommy-podcast/id1386673238.

Sandoz, Elizabeth. "Miraculous Mamas with Elizabeth Sandoz." https://podcasts.apple .com/us/podcast/miraculous-mamas/id1343507855.

Schulte, Lara, and Jenn Rout. "Generation.Mom with Laura & Jenn." https://podcasts .apple.com/us/podcast/generation-mom/id1399768538.

Tenety, Liz, and Motherly. "The Motherly Podcast." https://podcasts.apple.com/us /podcast/the-motherly-podcast/id1449924733.

Websites

- www.plussizebirth.com
- www.pelvicguru.com
- www.motherhood-understood.com
- www.thebluedotproject.com

Instagram Must-Follows

- @the.vagina.whisperer
- @getmomstrong
- @stopcensoringmotherhood
- @mommy.labornurse
- @scarymommy
- @empoweredbirthproject
- @birthwithoutfear
- @kids.eat.in.color
- @feedinglittles
- @busytoddler
- @plussizebirth

- @motherhoodunderstood
- @thebluedotprj
- @fatpositivefertility
- @mother.ly
- @thebirthhour
- @plusmommy
- @miraculousmamas
- @catandnat
- @goodmoms_badchoices
- @thatsinappropriate
- @generation.mom

BODY-POSITIVE FITNESS

Apps

"Joyn—Joyful Movement." Joyn. York64, 2020. apps.apple.com/us/app/joyn-joyful
-movement/id1471026020.

"The Underbelly Yoga." Underbelly. Fearless, 2020. apps.apple.com/us/app/the
-underbelly/id1446751733.

"Slow AF Run Club." Inspired Moments, 2020. apps.apple.com/us/app/slow-af-run-club
/id1494080105.

"Work It with MG." Madalin Giorgetta Fitness, 2020. apps.apple.com/us/app/work-it
-with-mg/id1444376673.

Website

- www.superfithero.com/pages/body-positive-fitness-finder

Podcast

- The Thick Thighs Save Lives Podcast

Instagram Must-Follows

- @iamchrissyking
- @decolonizing_fitness
- @laurenleavellfitness
- @carolynviggh
- @kanoagreene
- @300poundsandrunning
- @deadlifts_and_redlips
- @rozthediva
- @taralaferrara
- @mynameisjessamyn
- @themirnavator
- @iamlshauntay

- @fatgirlshiking
- @girlswhopowerlift
- @sistersofpowerlifting
- @letsjoyn
- @theunderbellyyoga
- @runslowaf
- @workitwithmg
- fatbabesmovement
- moritsummers
- shwpowerlifting
- autonomymovement
- thegirlgonestrong

Acknowledgments

This book was something I once dreamt of writing, and it was absolutely made possible because of the following people who guided me, encouraged me, and believed in my wild dreams.

MOM, DAD: For spending the last thirty years trusting me and allowing me the room to grow into the woman I am today. For being a constant soundboard to all my ideas and hyping up every single one of them.

MERRY, DIEHL: For all the moments you were so excited to spend hours upon hours with Maci while I wrote this book throughout all hours of the night. You have both been such a blessing in my life.

MANUEL, MARCUS, TILLY: For always being supportive from miles and miles away.

CAT: For listening to this dream of mine and pouring us a second mule to cheers an ultimate manifestation.

MY ENTIRE TEAM AT SIMON & SCHUSTER AND TILLER PRESS: For believing in me and my message enough to push and challenge me toward a goal that I never even thought possible. Especially my editor, Ronnie Alvarado, who was confident in this book from the moment we first spoke about it. And to Patrick Sullivan, for designing a beautiful cover. I am incredibly proud to be part of such a wonderful team of talented and passionate people.

ANGELA AND MY TEAM AT BLOGIST: For listening to every single one of my dreams and doing everything possible to make it happen.

STEPHANIE: For illustrating your magic into this book.

ASHLEY, AARONICA, DESIREE: For sharing your powerful stories without hesitation. I am forever inspired by your authenticity and desire to change the world.

EMILY: For all of our long voice texts during each of our breakdowns. You're a light in this world.

SHANE: For introducing me to powerlifting and teaching me how to lift. And for the beard. It's really cool.

UNDER ARMOUR: For inviting me to your Human Performance Summit and giving me the opportunity to prove that fat athletes are just as badass.

TARA: For your fierce passion for fitness and inclusivity. And giving me the best tips.

EVELYN TRIBOLE, CHRISTY HARRISON, LAURA THOMAS, CAROLINE DOONER: For writing books that completely changed my life during a time that life didn't quite feel worth living.

THE FAT ACCEPTANCE COMMUNITY: For showing the hell up before it was cool and creating space for fat women and humans like me to thrive at any and every capacity. It is because of women before me like Megan Jayne Crabbe, Sonya Renee Taylor, Virgie Tovar, Jes Baker, and Jessamyn Stanley who made it possible for women like me to experience the kind of self-confidence I experienced in the years that eventually led up to this book.

MACI: For being my sunshine.

BOBBY: For loving me before I ever learned to love myself. For all of the times you sat next to me on the bathroom floor as I cried in the bathtub. For every panic attack you approached calmly and understandingly. For your humor, your patience, your sexiness, and your reach-for-the-stars, over-the-fence, world-series kind of love.

Notes

1. "Beauty Redefined." Beauty Redefined. http://www.beautyredefined.org/.

2. Christy Harrison, "What Does Anti-Diet Really Mean?," www.christyharrision.com, December 18, 2018. https://christyharrison.com/blog/what-does-anti-diet-really-mean.

3. Joslyn P. Smith, "LIVE Well Act, Why It's Important," *NEDA Blog*, 2019, https://www .nationaleatingdisorders.org/blog/live-well-act-why-its-important.

4. R. M. Puhl, T. Andreyeva, and K. D. Brownell, "Perceptions of Weight Discrimination: Prevalence and Comparison to Race and Gender Discrimination in America," *International Journal of Obesity* (London) 32(6) (2008): 992–1000.

5. Thomas F. Cash and Linda Smolak, *Body Image: A Handbook of Science, Practice, and Prevention*, 2nd ed. (New York: Guilford Press, 2011).

6. Jeanne B. Martin, "The Development of Ideal Body Image Perceptions in the United States," *Nutrition Today* 45(3) (2010): 98–110.

7. T. Andreyeva, R. M. Puhl, K. D. Brownell, "Changes in Perceived Weight Discrimination among Americans, 1995–1996 through 2004–2006," *Obesity* (Silver Spring, MD) 16(5) (2008): 1129–34.

8. F. Grodstein et al., "Three-Year Follow-Up of Participants in a Commercial Weight Loss Program: Can You Keep It Off?," *Archives of Internal Medicine* 156(12) (1996): 1302–6; and D. Neumark-Sztainer et al., "Why Does Dieting Predict Weight Gain in Adolescents? Findings from Project EAT-II: A 5-Year Longitudinal Study," *Journal of the American Dietetic Association* 107(3) (2007): 448–55.

9. E. Wertheim, S. Paxton, and S. Blaney, "Body Image in Girls," in *Body Image, Eating Disorders, and Obesity in Youth: Assessment, Prevention, and Treatment*, 2nd ed., ed. L. Smolak and J. K. Thompson (Washington, DC: American Psychological Association, 2009), 47–76.

10. R. Hobbs et al., "How Adolescent Girls Interpret Weight-Loss Advertising," *Health Education Research* 21(5) (2006): 719–30.

11. Evelyn Tribole, "Definition of Intuitive Eating," Original Intuitive Eating Pros, July 17, 2019, https://www.intuitiveeating.org/definition-of-intuitive-eating/; and Evelyn Tribole and Elyse Resch, *Intuitive Eating: A Revolutionary Program That Works*, 3rd ed. (New York: St. Martin's Griffin, 2012).

12. V. Grigorescu, T. Comeaux Plowden, and L. Pal, "Polycystic Ovary Syndrome," Office on Women's Health, April 1, 2019, https://www.womenshealth.gov/a-z-topics /polycystic-ovary-syndrome.

13. M. Perales, R. Artal, and A. Lucia, "Exercise During Pregnancy," *JAMA* 317(11) (2017): 1113–14.

14. World Health Organization, *Mental Health Aspects of Women's Reproductive Health: A Global Review of the Literature* (Geneva, Switzerland: World Health Organization, 2009).

15. B. N. Gaynes et al., "Perinatal Depression: Prevalence, Screening Accuracy, and Screening Outcomes," *Evidence Report / Technological Assessment (Summary)* 119 (2005): 1–8.

16. K. L. Wisner, B. L. Parry, and C. M. Piontek, "Clinical Practice. Postpartum Depression," *New England Journal of Medicine* 347(3) (2002): 194–99.

17. C. D. Mathers and D. Loncar, "Projections of Global Mortality and Burden of Disease from 2002 to 2030," *PLoS Medicine* 3(11) (2006): e442.

18. R. Cantwell, T. Clutton-Brock, and G. Cooper, "Saving Mothers' Lives: Reviewing Maternal Deaths to Make Motherhood Safer: 2006–2008," *BJOG* 122(5) (April 2015): e1.

19. V. Lindahl, J. L. Pearson, and L. Colpe, "Prevalence of Suicidality during Pregnancy and the Postpartum," *Archives of Women's Mental Health* 8(2) (2005): 77–87.

20. R. C. Boyd et al., "Screening and Referral for Postpartum Depression among Low-Income Women: A Qualitative Perspective from Community Health Workers," *Depression Research and Treatment*, 2011, https://doi.org/10.1155/2011/320605.

21. Dove Self-Esteem Project, 2017, https://www.dove.com/us/en/dove-self-esteem -project.html.

22. S. L. Watson et al., "High-Intensity Resistance and Impact Training Improves Bone Mineral Density and Physical Function in Postmenopausal Women with Osteopenia and Osteoporosis: The LIFTMOR Randomized Controlled Trial," *Journal of Bone and Mineral Research* 33(2) (2018): 211–20; published correction appears in *Journal of Bone and Mineral Research* 34(3) (March 2019): 572.

23. J. Grgic, E. T. Trexler, and B. Lazinica, "Effects of Caffeine Intake on Muscle Strength and Power: A Systematic Review and Meta-analysis," *Journal of the International Society of Sports Nutrition*, 2018.

24. J. D. Bosse and B. M. Dixon, "Dietary Protein to Maximize Resistance Training: A Review and Examination of Protein Spread and Change Theories," *Journal of the International Society of Sports Nutrition*, 2012.

25. Derave et al., "Beta-Alanine Supplementation Augments Muscle Carnosine Content and Attenuates Fatigue during Repeated Isokinetic Contraction Bouts in Trained Sprinters," *Journal of Applied Physiology* 103(5) (2007): 1736–43, originally published 1985; and R. B. Kreider, D. S. Kalman, and J. Antonio, "International Society of Sports Nutrition Position Stand: Safety and Efficacy of Creatine Supplementation in Exercise, Sport, and Medicine," *Journal of the International Society of Sports Nutrition* 14(1) (2017): 18.

About the Author

MEG BOGGS is a mother, wife, content creator, powerlifter, and self-empowerment advocate who has made it her mission to help women embrace their insecurities. Meg first took to her blog and Instagram to share her journey through motherhood, revealing her postpartum body through a series of emotionally raw posts that earned her attention from moms and global media, including CNN, *Good Morning America*, and *People*. With advocacy of issues from mental health awareness to fitness inclusivity, promoted alongside body-positive imagery on all of her social media platforms, Meg continues to spark discourse about fat bodies and the experiences of plus-size women. She lives with her family in Fort Worth, Texas. Follow her on Instagram @Meg.Boggs, TikTok @Meg.Boggs, and online at MegBoggs.com.